DATE DUE

AVON PUBLIC LIBRARY
BOX 977 / 200 BENCHMARK RD.
AVON, COLORADO 81620

Health Trackers

How Technology is Helping Us Monitor and Improve Our Health

Richard MacManus

ROWMAN & LITTLEFIELD
Lanham • Boulder • New York • London

ADVANCE REVIEWS FOR *TRACKERS*

Few writers have the technical savvy and trend-spotting abilities to capture and document the rapidly changing digital health technology landscape.

Dr. Indu Subaiya
Co-chairman & CEO, Health 2.0

This book is a great overview of the world of self-trackers ... With insights from enthusiasts, patients, doctors and self-tracking companies, this book provides a well-researched and highly readable analysis of the field. I'd recommend this book to anyone interested in using smartphones, activity monitors or even the new Apple Watch to help them manage their health.

Dr. Chris Paton
Clinical Researcher, Health Informatics
University of Oxford, UK

Richard MacManus has penned a must-read book both for anyone looking to get or stay healthy and the millions of care givers working to help them on that journey.... Trackers is that rare treat of a technology book that manages to stay current despite a fast-moving news cycle, and succeeds at offering its lucky readers a peek at what's next.

Brian Dolan
Editor & co-founder, *MobiHealthNews*

This book will be a wake-up call to health services and health researchers about the rapidly approaching importance of patient-reported data and the opportunities for collaborating with the medical establishment.

Dr. Robyn Whittaker
Public health physician & health researcher
Waitemata District Health Board & University of Auckland, NZ

Richard MacManus' new book Trackers *is an insightful, very personal look at how health tracking technology is changing the human condition.*

Amy Tenderich
Founder & editor, diabetesmine.com

MacManus combines his position as a leading technology pundit with the story of his own personal health journey, to give us insightful pointers towards the future of healthcare.

Mike Kirkwood
CTO, QxMD Inc

What we call "quantified self" today will become the medicine of tomorrow. If you want to catch a glimpse of what medicine in the coming century will look like, Trackers *is a must-read . . . Richard MacManus weaves masterful storytelling with a passion driven by his own health challenges. This isn't just a book about self-tracking, it's a book about the future of health.*

Leonard Kish
MSIS/MBA, MS Biomedical Sciences,
Principal & co-founder at VivaPhi, author at HL7Standards.com

This is a must-read book. It ventures out onto the edge of healthcare and helps us to understand how technology is giving us much more data about our physical condition. . . . We're in the very early stages of a big shift in healthcare and MacManus helps to see where we need to go from here. Our health depends on it.

John Hagel
Co-chairman, Center for the Edge & author, *The Power of Pull*

I feel like I learned something about myself just by reading it . . . and I'm supposed to know it all already!

Buster Benson
Product Manager, Twitter

This book helps us see not only who we are but who we can be with technology.

Brian Solis
Digital analyst & author of *What's the Future of Business*

Published by Rowman & Littlefield
A wholly owned subsidary of The Rowman & Littlefield Publishing Group, Inc.
4501 Forbes Boulevard, Suite 200, Lanham, Maryland 20706
www.rowman.com

Unit A, Whitacre Mews, 26-34 Stannary Street, London SE11 4AB

Copyright © 2015 by Richard McManus & David Bateman Ltd.

First published in 2015 by
David Bateman Ltd.
30 Tarndale Grove
Albany, Auckland 1330
New Zealand

All rights reserved. No part of this book may be reproduced in any form or
by any electronic or mechanical means, including information storage and
retrieval systems, without written permission from the publisher, except by a
reviewer who may quote passages in a review.

British Library Cataloguing in Publication Information Available

Library of Congress Cataloging-in-Publication Data Available

ISBN 978-1-4422-5355-1 (cloth : alk. paper) — ISBN 978-1-4422-5356-8
(electronic)

♾™ The paper used in this publication meets the minimum requirements of
American National Standard for Information Sciences—Permanence of Paper
for Printed Library Materials, ANSI/NISO Z39.48-1992.

Printed in the United States of America

CONTENTS

Acknowledgments   7

Introduction   9

Chapter One
Buster Benson's self-tracking odyssey   23

Chapter Two
The pedometer on steroids: tracking activity with Fitbit   41

Chapter Three
Diet wars: tracking food with MyFitnessPal   59

Chapter Four
The tao of weight tracking   78

Chapter Five
How useful is genetics? Me & my 23andMe results   96

Chapter Six
Inception: tracking the brain   115

Chapter Seven
Bacteria nation: tracking the microbiome with uBiome   128

Chapter Eight
The health dashboard: TicTrac   147

Chapter Nine
The modern doctor: Dr. Robin Berzin   166

Chapter Ten
Tracking + medicine: MD Revolution   184

Epilogue   202

The author   218

Further reading & references   219

Index   221

ACKNOWLEDGMENTS

It's strange to thank a disease, but I must say that getting type 1 diabetes in November 2007 was my major inspiration for writing this book. It made me realize how fragile the human body is and how crucial it is to look after it. Becoming a diabetic also makes one realize the importance of a loving family. So I'm grateful to my parents Kevin and Judy, and my daughter Rosabelle, for their continued love and support.

I started my technology blog ReadWriteWeb in April 2003 and left it in October 2012 to begin research for this book. In the nine and a half years I spent building ReadWrite (as it's now called), I made a great many friends, especially within my own company, whose many writers and other staff over the years inspired and motivated me as a technology journalist. I also met a lot of smart and talented people outside my company, via the international blogosphere, and it still amazes me that anyone can now build a media entity that is read all over the world. For that I thank one of my personal heroes, Sir Tim Berners-Lee, for creating the World Wide Web. I met Sir Tim in 2009, to interview him for ReadWrite. It was one of the proudest moments in my life.

I'm very grateful to all of the entrepreneurs and medical professionals I interviewed for this book. Every one of them was very passionate about the potential of technology to improve healthcare. I'd also like to thank the organizers of the Health 2.0 Conference, the Personalized Medicine World Conference, and the Quantified Self Silicon Valley Meetup Group.

Last but not least, my heartfelt appreciation goes to all of the forward-thinking doctors in the world, in particular my own doctor, Dr. Tony Crutchley of the Thorndon Medical Centre in Wellington, New Zealand. Dr. Crutchley has been my GP since 2000 and has guided me through the highs and lows of my own health. Although I'm a firm believer in the value of technology to help me monitor my health, I will always rely on my doctor for his expertise and humanity. I hope everyone who reads this book feels the same way about their family doctor.

Richard MacManus, October 2014

INTRODUCTION

My interest in health technology was triggered by a visit to my doctor's office on November 19, 2007. That was when I found out I had diabetes. Looking back on it today, it's remarkable how ignorant I was about the state of my own body at the time. In the weeks leading up to that doctor's visit, I'd known something was wrong with my health. There were warning signs—I was rapidly losing weight and feeling increasingly irritable with my family and friends. But I did my best to ignore it and just get on with life. Like many men, I didn't want to show weakness. I was busy. I ran a stressful startup, and I had a young family to support. So I didn't have time to worry; my health was the least of my concerns ... or at least, that was my mindset in 2007.

I don't recall when I first noticed the symptoms of diabetes, but it was a short holiday I had with my wife and six-year-old daughter at the end of September 2007 that signaled something wasn't right. We'd taken the Cook Strait ferry from Wellington City, at the bottom of New Zealand's North Island, to the seaport town of Picton at the top of the South Island. Our destination was Kaikoura, a scenic coastal town a couple of hours' drive from Picton. On the way we visited my grandmother in Blenheim, about midway between Picton and Kaikoura. I couldn't have known it then, but it was to be the last time I'd see her—she died unexpectedly just over a month later.

After leaving Blenheim to drive to Kaikoura, I began to feel strange. I had developed an unquenchable thirst! I'd bought some power drinks for the journey, but I was rapidly going through them, guzzling whole bottles in one go. Funnily enough, it wasn't the thirst that concerned me. It was that I wanted to pee every ten minutes. OK, I was drinking a lot of fluids, but surely it's not normal to have to pee so often? I can usually "hold it in" for much longer than that, I said to myself—somewhat shamefully. In hindsight, that reaction was more evidence of my macho sensibility around health. In fact, it was the sugar in those power drinks that made my body want to pee so quickly. It wasn't a personal failure to hold it in, because with diabetes the body simply can't cope with large amounts of glucose. So it does the logical thing: makes you get rid of it through peeing. Of course at the time I had no clue that this was a symptom of diabetes. It just felt like an alien had taken over my body and for some reason it didn't like fluids.

It was a cloudy day and spots of rain had started to fall as I clambered out of the car for the umpteenth time to find a tree or bush to relieve myself behind. The east coast of the South Island is rugged, beautiful territory. On the drive to Kaikoura we'd seen the wild blue of the Pacific Ocean to our left, the white spittle of sea foam whipping up in the wind onto the highway. On our right was miles of green countryside. It was gorgeous scenery, but I wasn't enjoying it in the least. The alien inside me just wanted to pee all the time, so all I could think about in the car was finding the next place to stop. There were other signs that I wasn't feeling right. I was flushed and bad-tempered and I argued with my wife. I felt agitated, but I put it down to a combination of the strange peeing frenzy, together with the business stress I was under at that time.

Those were heady times for me. In 2007 I ran a technology blog and in that year business was ramping up quickly. In September I'd hired my second staff writer. There were now several of us writing the blog on a daily basis. But I was juggling much more than writing, as my diary from that time shows. I was doing everything from selling ads, to managing employees and contractors, getting the website redesigned, organizing the accounts, and much more. In short I was your typical bootstrapped entrepreneur, harried and wearing too many hats. The strain was starting to show.

Despite the obvious signs of physical and emotional distress I'd noticed on the Kaikoura trip, it wasn't till a week after I'd returned from holiday that I made an appointment with my doctor. I finally went to see him on October 10. I remember that he mentioned diabetes as a possible diagnosis, but that he wouldn't know for sure until I did some blood tests. He gave me a signed slip of paper to take to the blood clinic. I should have gone straight away, but incredibly I decided to leave it till I got back from an upcoming overseas business trip. I simply put the possible diabetes diagnosis out of my mind. I didn't even do any research on what this might mean for my health.

On October 14, I flew for twelve hours across the Pacific to San Francisco. I was attending a couple of technology events: a one-day smaller event called Mobile 2.0 and a larger three-day conference called the Web 2.0 Summit. It was on this trip that I bought my first iPhone. The smartphone revolution was just beginning in 2007 and, as a technology blogger, I was right in the middle of it. In the coming years the iPhone and similar mobile devices would have a huge impact on healthcare. But I'm getting ahead of myself. At that time, 2007, I was barely interested in my own health—let alone the healthcare system. I was only interested in playing with this shiny new gadget I'd bought. On October 23, I arrived back in New Zealand. Work and playing with my iPhone were still clearly more important than my own health, because for another couple of weeks I continued to put off the blood test that my doctor had requested.

Then my grandmother in Blenheim died. We went back to the South Island for her funeral. It was that trip that finally persuaded me to look into my own health. I remember in particular the ferry ride back. It was the worst I'd ever been on, with foul weather and rough seas lurching the ferry up and down. I got terribly seasick and spent much of the time hogging—and hugging—one of the ship's toilets. Perhaps this experience, the funeral of my grandmother and my extreme seasickness, made me more aware of the vagaries of life and health. So I finally did the blood test and made a follow-up appointment with my doctor.

Nothing could have prepared me for what the doctor told me on Monday, November 19, 2007. He usually has a kindly, amused expression on his face, but this time he looked serious. "I'm sorry to say this, old boy," he said, "but you have diabetes."

I didn't even know what diabetes was at that time, let alone that there were two distinct types. My doctor confessed that he too wasn't sure if it was type 1 or type 2. I'd need further tests to find out. Type 2 is the far more common one, making up 85–90% of all diabetes patients. It's when the body still produces insulin—specifically, your pancreas does—but the insulin doesn't do the job it's supposed to: regulate your blood sugar levels. Type 2 is typically associated with being overweight, because that puts strain on your body and can lead to problems absorbing the insulin from the pancreas. I had been overweight a bit, in the way that many men in their mid-thirties add a paunch around their tummies through bad diet. So it was possible I had type 2. But more likely I was type 1, even though it's rare to get it in your thirties. The common name for type 1 used to be juvenile diabetes, because it's most common in children.

About a week later, a specialist confirmed that I had type 1. It's an autoimmune disease, I discovered, in which the body's immune system mistakenly attacks the insulin-producing cells in the pancreas. Your immune system kills off those cells, so your body can no longer produce the insulin it needs.

There is no known reason for getting type 1 diabetes, especially in your thirties. I would discover later that I had a tiny genetic predisposition to it. But it was such a small risk that there had to be a trigger in my environment. Probably the business and personal stress I was under in 2007 was part of it, although a completely random virus could have been the main cause. Regardless, that doctor's visit on November 19 was a huge wake-up call for me. My body no longer performed one of its basic functions: producing insulin to control blood sugar levels. So I would have to inject insulin every day for the rest of my life. I would have to forever closely monitor what I eat and drink. I would—finally—have to pay attention to my daily health.

Surprisingly, I sounded relatively upbeat on Twitter later on that fateful day. Here's how I summed up my new health status on November 19, 2007, in 140 characters or less: "Discovered today, from doctor, I have Diabetes! So no more sugar and beer for me. Glad I found out about it now tho, can control it now." Little did I know then that the digital world—and in particular smartphones—would play a crucial part in helping me achieve a level of control over my diabetes.

A changed man

"How are you doing, old boy?" inquired my doctor jovially. He turned to his PC and clicked through several screens until he found the store of medical data that had my name on it. It was early July 2013 and I was here for my annual diabetic checkup. The last time I'd been to see my doctor was a year ago, for my previous checkup.

I'd made some significant changes to my healthcare since then. I'd begun a low-carb diet in March 2013, which had improved my ability to control my blood sugar levels—the key marker for diabetes management. That change in diet had allowed me to reduce the amount of insulin I took every day. So on this visit I was looking forward to sharing my new formula for managing diabetes. The doctor had noticed my upbeat mood and also spotted the iPad I'd carried into his office. "You've got something to show me?" he asked, genuinely curious.

Traditionally, the relationship you have with your family doctor is a paternalistic one. You do an annual medical checkup, after which you're sat down in the doctor's office and given a sanitized version of your health profile. "You're doing just fine, but keep an eye on your blood pressure," your doctor might tell you. But now we're moving into a world where we are taking responsibility for our own health, or at least for the measurement and regular monitoring of key health data. This was what I was about to show my doctor.

I swiped open the iPad on my lap. Inside this magical device I had a year's worth of data about my own health. Paramount among the data horde was my daily blood glucose readings, the results of pinpricks to my fingers that I do about five or six times a day. That data was sitting in a spreadsheet, augmented by various graphs I'd created to map the trends.

The original data had been input into an iPhone app called Diamedic. I'd shown my doctor this spreadsheet a year ago too. But this year I was armed with much more data. I had a separate spreadsheet that logged the foods I'd eaten over a period of a couple of months. That was from an iPhone app called MyFitnessPal.

Another spreadsheet featured a few months of daily activity data—how many steps I took every day. That came from a pedometer device called the Fitbit One. I also had a year's worth of weight readings, courtesy of an Internet-connected scale called the Fitbit Aria. Finally, I had a copy of my genetic profile displayed on my iPad, via a personal genomics company called 23andMe.

What I'd been doing over the past year is known as self-tracking. I had measured and monitored a number of different data points about my body: the foods I ate in a day, how many steps I took, how much I weighed, my blood glucose readings. I could have added other data points, had I wanted to. My heart rate, my emotions and moods, even brain scans. All of this can be tracked now, through the use of Internet-connected applications and devices.

My doctor sidled his chair up next to mine so that he could examine all this information on my iPad. None of it replaced what he has on his own computer screen. I would still have to undergo the blood tests and other examinations that my doctor does every year to track how my diabetes is doing. Indeed, I would love to have on my iPad the same information that my doctor has access to on his PC. The best he can do currently is give me a printout of the main readings, which he does every time I visit him. Nevertheless, the data I've collected about my own body over the past year and stored on my iPad gives me a sense of control over my health and wellness that I didn't have before. It complements the data my doctor has.

The rise of tracking apps and devices

As with most new forms of technology, self-tracking originated in Silicon Valley, where to this day it goes by the geeky term "quantified self." The idea of quantified self is to measure aspects of yourself. Some of these things I'll be describing in this book, things like tracking how many steps you take in a day, how many calories you consume and use up, your weight over time. The term quantified self was coined in 2007 by two editors at *Wired* magazine, Gary Wolf and Kevin Kelly. The pair defined it as "a collaboration of users and tool makers who share an interest in self-knowledge through self-tracking." The founding principle, wrote Kelly in an October 2007 blog post, was this: "Unless something can be measured, it cannot be improved."

To familiarize myself with the latest quantified self trends, in January 2013 I attended a meeting of the Quantified Self Silicon Valley Meetup Group. It was held at the San Jose head office of IT consultancy Accenture. San Jose is about a 45-minute drive south from San Francisco. It's the largest city in Silicon Valley and the home of many software and IT companies. The head offices of Cisco, Netgear, and Fry's Electronics are all in San Jose. This is old-school Silicon Valley, but new ideas are as likely to germinate in San Jose as in Palo Alto just up the road. The Quantified Self Silicon Valley Meetup was founded at the end of 2010 and has about 1,000 members, many of them the engineers and programmers who work at companies like Cisco and Netgear. It's a very technical group whose members are also likely to attend the Silicon Valley Android Developers Meetup, the Bay Area useR Group (for adherents of the R programing language), and the SF Bayarea Machine Learning Meetup.

That evening I saw presentations from a young man who tracked the quality of his sleep (he had a disorder called sleep apnea), a man who tracked and categorized every single activity in his day in order to be more self-aware, and a businessman who had invented a body-scanning device that looked like an airport security machine. There were other presentations, including one from the subject of Chapter Four of this book: weight tracker Amelia Greenhall. All the presentations were at the cutting edge of self-tracking—highly technical and outside the norm. But if there's one thing I've learned as a long-time analyst of Silicon Valley technology, it's that the best of it eventually filters down to the rest of us. Over time technology gets less geeky, more practical, and easier to use. That's precisely what's happening right now with self-tracking, thanks to smartphones and new gadgets such as the Apple Watch.

> **Over time technology gets less geeky, more practical, and easier to use.**

It all started with the iPhone launch in mid-2007, although it would be a good couple of years after that before health apps made an impact. When I bought my first iPhone in October 2007, like every other geek at the time I looked on it as a shiny new toy to play with. When you think of the iPhone now, or indeed any smartphone, you immediately think of "apps"—third-party software applications such as the photo service Instagram or music player Spotify. But there were no official apps for the iPhone in 2007. Apple's now famous App Store, which enables you to install third-party apps onto the iPhone, didn't arrive until July 2008. In 2007 the iPhone relied on so-called "Mobile Web" sites, which were miniature versions of websites that ran on the iPhone's Safari browser. But these early mobile websites were not very interactive. So it wasn't until mid- to late 2008 that mobile apps began to be developed and released. They weren't just for the iPhone at that point either. The first Android smartphone arrived on the scene in October 2008. Android is an open-source mobile platform originally designed by Google. Today it rivals the iPhone as the most popular smartphone platform.

There were a smattering of health apps released on the App Store in July 2008. One of the earliest was called iCalorie and was added to the App Store in mid-July of that year for $4.99. Developed by a one-man-shop software developer in Tampa, Florida, the app was very basic. All it offered was an interface to input your calories and the app would then add up the daily total. It failed to set the App Store alight. As one harsh reviewer put it at the time, "no food and nutrition label database makes it completely useless." Despite being fast off the blocks in the App Store, iCalorie stalled and stopped releasing updates in August 2008. Its failure signaled that smartphone users were not going to put up with unsophisticated apps.

It took well over a year for better health apps to come onto the market. If iCalorie was an anemic app, the MyFitnessPal iPhone app released in December 2009 was a much healthier specimen. Unlike its weak calorie-counting cousin, the MyFitnessPal iPhone app was loaded with data muscle. After launching its website back in September 2005, MyFitnessPal had spent the following four years methodically building up a weighty database of food—not just of calories, but counts of carbohydrates, protein, saturated fat, and other food data. So when MyFitnessPal finally released a smartphone app at the end of 2009, users were impressed with the wide selection of food items in the database. It made it so much easier for people to input their calorie data. MyFitnessPal saw an immediate surge in popularity after the iPhone app was released, because for the first time its users were able to track their food on the go. It's no coincidence that the release of the smartphone app was, in hindsight, the tipping point for MyFitnessPal. It's now the dominant online calorie counter on the market. We'll delve into that success story in Chapter Three.

After 2009, many other sophisticated and increasingly easier to use smartphone apps for health became available. But it wasn't just smartphones that pushed along self-tracking. New Web-connected devices were being cautiously released in 2009 and curious geeks were quick to try them out.

One of the most popular of these new-fangled tracking devices was from a startup called Fitbit, the subject of Chapter Two. Fitbit's self-styled "pedometer on steroids" was a small rectangular device that you clipped onto your belt or bra. It enabled you to track the number of steps you took in a day. While pedometers were not new—such devices have a history going back to the 18th century—the Fitbit was much more precise than traditional pedometers, plus it uploaded the data to the Internet. The first Fitbit tracker was launched in September 2009, just a few months before MyFitnessPal's iPhone app. Also released in the US in September 2009 was the Withings scale, an Internet-connected weight scale that we will look at in Chapter Four.

These new smartphone apps and tracking devices were putting people in control of their day-to-day health data for the first time. Now you could track and store on the Internet what you ate, how much activity you did in a day, your weight readings, and more. At about the same time all this was happening, personal genomics burst onto the scene. As fate would have it, the very day that my doctor informed me that I had diabetes (November 19, 2007) was also the day that 23andMe officially launched. For the first time, 23andMe was offering a direct-to-consumer DNA test. The price was steep at first, at $1,000. But by the end of 2012, 23andMe had dropped the price below $100 in a bid to reach its stated goal of one million customers.

Many people still have qualms about doing a DNA test. Do you really want to know your risk of getting a disease like type 1 diabetes, which isn't something you can prevent? Another problem that 23andMe has faced since its launch is that genetic results are probabilistic, not deterministic. In other words, you have a percentage risk factor for any given disease. The trouble is, the scientific community still knows very little about how genes contribute to our daily health and wellbeing. So your results could be very misleading. In many cases, the environment you live in is a far more important factor in contracting a disease than your genetic makeup.

When I finally did the 23andMe test in 2012, I discovered that I had four times the average risk of getting type 1 diabetes. But that risk was still only 4.1%. In other words, if I lived my life 100 times, I'd probably only get type 1 diabetes in four of those lifetimes. I was just unlucky to get it in this particular lifetime. Indeed, according to the latest medical theory about how type 1 diabetes is contracted, the main factor may have been a rogue virus—something I couldn't have either predicted or prevented.

So the usefulness of genetic testing is debatable. We'll explore those controversies, together with the known benefits of getting your DNA tested, in Chapter Five.

Whatever the challenges in interpreting your 23andMe results, there is a general shift happening in the healthcare system toward people taking control of their health data. Genomics is a key part of that shift. It doesn't get more personal than knowing the makeup of your own DNA, what 23andMe co-founder and CEO Anne Wojcicki calls "the digital manifestation of you." Wojcicki is proud of the fact that you don't need a doctor's prescription to get a DNA test. Her goal is to let people assess their own chances of contracting diseases and modify their lifestyles if they think it's necessary. Traditionally, of course, that's been the role of your doctor. "The paternalism of the medical industry is insane," Wojcicki told *Marie Claire* magazine in 2010, "but scientific advances are changing all that. It's not their world anymore. We're taking it back."

A new type of healthcare

It doesn't have to be as combative as 23andMe's Anne Wojcicki makes out. My own doctor is open-minded about the health data that I track about myself and he was curious to check it out on my iPad during my recent visit. You'll also see in this book that modern doctors are adopting tools like 23andMe too. In Chapter Nine you'll meet Dr. Robin Berzin, a young doctor in New York City who is incorporating data from sources like 23andMe and Fitbit into her daily practice. Dr. Berzin sees the ultimate doctor-patient relationship as more of a collaboration than a consultation. The doctor is the medical expert, that hasn't changed. But Berzin recognizes that patients are bringing a lot more of their health data to the table now.

The corollary of we patients having more control over our health data is that the onus is on us to take responsibility for it. If we have more data at our fingertips—everything from our DNA data to Fitbit—then we have the opportunity to use it to try to prevent disease. There's a term for this: preventative medicine. Western medicine up till now has tended to be reactive; you get sick, so you go to the doctor or hospital. The job of the doctor is to assess your symptoms and then try to cure you. But if you can prevent disease from occurring in the first place, wouldn't that be a better way to practice medicine? That approach is gaining traction, thanks in part to self-tracking and personal genomics.

It's important to note that preventative medicine isn't a panacea. This approach to healthcare has its limits, at this point in time. It all depends on what disease we're talking about. Type 1 diabetes probably cannot be headed off at the pass, but type 2 diabetes definitely can be. If your DNA shows an increased risk of type 2 and your MyFitnessPal and Fitbit data shows that you consume far more calories than you use up every day, then those are powerful signals for you to take preventative measures to try to stop type 2 before it hits. Indeed, it's relatively easy to prevent type 2 if you are forearmed with the data and the willpower to make changes to your lifestyle. Other diseases are much harder to stop. There has been no bigger, or more chilling, example of this in modern medicine than cancer. It was the scourge of the 20th century and continues to be into the 21st century. In his groundbreaking book *The Emperor of All Maladies: A Biography of Cancer*, Siddhartha Mukherjee wrote that cancer is a disease characterized by "uncontrollable pathological cell division." So there's a limit to what we can control, even in this new age of preventative medicine.

Self-tracking has the potential to lead to remarkable insights about the human body.

Even so, self-tracking has the potential to lead to remarkable insights about the human body. Every era has its diseases that hit large swathes of the population. The main ones of the early 21st century are cancer, heart disease, autoimmune diseases (such as type 1 diabetes), and diseases related to dysfunction in our bodies (such as type 2 diabetes). What all of these otherwise disparate diseases have in common is that they hit us from *within* whereas, prior to the 20th century, the most virulent diseases were those that attacked our bodies from *without*: tuberculosis, flu epidemics, plagues. Back in the 19th century, you could do very little to prevent being struck down with a disease like tuberculosis—which literally traveled through the air, via people sneezing or coughing. But the fact that modern diseases strike from within our own bodies gives us a glimmer of hope. With tools like personal genomics and brain scans (covered in Chapter Six), you can now see inside your body. With self-tracking devices and apps, you can analyze your body's inputs and outputs. It's by no means a cure-all, but these technologies allow you to better understand your body and the impact of your lifestyle on it.

Having more health data is one thing, using it is quite another. Even in cases where there is a clear path to prevention, such as the signs of type 2 diabetes, it can be very difficult to implement the changes in your lifestyle necessary to prevent it. Currently in Silicon Valley there is a stampede to design the latest wearable gadget that helps you make lifestyle changes. We'll look at the Fitbit in Chapter Two, as an example of the current generation of wearables. But as uber tracker Buster Benson points out in Chapter One, merely having a device such as Fitbit isn't enough to make you want to use it. You have to want to make a big effort to change your existing behavior.

We'll explore behavior change fully throughout this book. In Chapter Four, we look at how self-tracking early adopter Amelia Greenhall has implemented her own custom weight loss program. In essence, she's had the self-discipline to make changes in her lifestyle based on her weight readings over the years. The alternative approach is to join an organization like Weight Watchers, which uses a social support system to encourage its members to make lifestyle changes to lose weight. I'll explore the differences between those two approaches in Chapter Four.

In the final analysis, self-tracking is about caring for your body. Tracking needn't be an obsessive thing, as it is for Buster Benson and (to a lesser degree) Amelia Greenhall.

Simply knowing more about your genetic makeup, through a 23andMe DNA test, and tracking your food and activity habits using tools like MyFitnessPal and Fitbit, can help you identify patterns in your body and lifestyle. What you do with that information is up to you.

You may be wondering if the medical establishment is joining the self-tracking revolution. Eventually they won't have a choice, but forward-thinking doctors are jumping into the fray now. I've already mentioned Dr. Robin Berzin, a practicing doctor in New York City and the subject of Chapter Nine. Dr. Berzin doesn't just prescribe drugs, she also prescribes self-tracking tools to her patients. In Chapter Ten you'll also meet Dr. Samir Damani, who straddles both the medical and technology worlds. He's a practicing cardiologist in the San Diego region, but he also runs a tracking startup called MD Revolution. As the name of his startup suggests, MD Revolution is bringing self-tracking tools into the doctor's office. Dr. Damani calls it a new form of medical service and likens it to joining a gym. You pay a monthly fee and get access to a mix of medical expertise and guidance in the use of self-tracking tools.

The healthcare revolution this book will describe isn't about the things you traditionally associate with the medical system. It's not about hospitals, health insurance, or drugs. Self-tracking is all about data—lots of it, and most of it under your control. Technology is driving this sea change in our healthcare system and it's all in service of you.

Are you ready to get personal about your health? Let's start by visiting a man who has been self-tracking since he was in high school.

CHAPTER ONE

BUSTER BENSON'S SELF-TRACKING ODYSSEY

We can change our behavior and habits (it requires a lot of energy).

Buster Benson, "My Beliefs"

Change has been a constant in the life of Buster Benson, a 36-year-old Web developer and serial entrepreneur from Seattle. He changes his behavior and habits often, in an ongoing quest to find a mix of daily activities that will make him happy. He regularly experiments with things like what to eat every day, how much quality time he spends with his young family, what's the right number of sit-ups to do (and when to do them), and how much time he spends doing rewarding work. In the name of change, Buster Benson has even gone so far as to change his name. Not once, but twice. A few years ago, Buster Benson was known as Buster McLeod. Before that he was Erik Benson, the name given to him by his parents. Change is what drives Buster Benson, although paradoxically his goal is to find an equilibrium of happiness in his life.

Benson's ongoing life changes have been recorded on the Internet since 1999. Some would say he's an obsessive self-tracker and ask why he puts so much personal data on the Web. But his compulsive need to change signifies an ongoing search for meaning in his life. As for why it's on the Internet, that's because technology offers him a way to easily track his personal data and connect it with other people.

The four main reasons to self-track

There are any number of reasons to self-track, but I've narrowed it down to four main ones. I myself only self-track for the first reason. I'd wager that most of you are the same; or perhaps you don't self-track at all right now. As for Buster Benson, he ticks all four boxes.

The first reason to self-track is to monitor and measure your health, to ensure that you're living a healthy lifestyle. This is by far the most common reason. As you'll discover in this book, a whole industry has cropped up to enable self-tracking for health purposes: everything from wristband pedometers like the Fitbit Flex and Nike FuelBand, to smart watches like Pebble and Apple Watch, to Internet-connected scales like the Withings scale, to mobile heart-rate monitors, to smartphone apps like MyFitnessPal. We will explore some of these gadgets and apps—and find out how effective they actually are—in upcoming chapters. In Benson's case, he's currently tracking his fitness with a Fitbit.

The second reason to self-track is to monitor your daily mood. Or to put it more grandly, to track your day-to-day happiness. The search for personal happiness has been a consistent theme in Buster Benson's self-tracking experiments. At one point he developed an online application called the "Morale-O-Meter" to help him track his moods.

The third reason to self-track is to improve yourself in some way, to become a better person. Don't worry, this isn't a self-help book—the self-help industry is already overloaded with self-styled gurus who are only too willing to be your guide. But how do you ensure that you stay on the straight and narrow? Self-tracking is one way to do that. For example, Buster Benson wants to be a better husband and father, so he aims to spend a certain amount of quality time each day with his wife and two-year-old son. He tracks his family time every day, in a spreadsheet, to help him be a better Buster.

The fourth reason to self-track is the least common. It's to track your search for the meaning of life. That sounds rather grand, but the fact is that everybody searches for meaning in their life. Sometimes it's a spiritual quest, but often it's a pragmatic one—like finding a career that is meaningful to you. What's unusual is to track this process over time, but that's precisely what Buster Benson is doing. He's posted his life goals to the Internet and even has a publicly accessible online document called "My Beliefs." He reflects on his goals and beliefs often, modifying and adding to the files whenever he's learned something new. All these changes are tracked on the Web.

So those are the four main reasons for self-tracking: 1) to track your health; 2) to track your mood; 3) to monitor a self-improvement goal; 4) to help you find meaning in your life. This book will focus mostly on the first goal, tracking for health purposes. Not only is that the most common form of self-tracking, it's also having huge ramifications for the healthcare industry. But before we explore health tracking, it's worthwhile taking a look at the other three reasons too—if only to see how far you can take the concept of self-tracking. This is where we turn back to Buster Benson.

Benson is an early adopter and more avid about self-tracking than most. However, it's important to note that he's not doing anything you or I wouldn't do. He's not an extreme self-tracker. He hasn't implanted a microchip in his body and he hasn't undertaken to record every living moment of his life online. He's not after a book deal or his own reality TV show. No, Buster Benson is quite normal underneath it all. He's a family man who tracks simple things about his life: how many sit-ups he does, how much time he spends with his family, what his career goals are. He isn't even that bothered by numbers, which you'd think he would be as a quantified-self fanatic. In fact much of what Benson tracks is recorded using a straightforward "true or false" question. Today I did ten sit-ups, true or false? Or, today I spent an hour with my son, true or false?

You may not see the need to emulate the amount of tracking that Benson does. Indeed, I'd recommend against it, as it's a lot of work! But we're all interested in monitoring our daily health and wellbeing. We all want to change something about ourselves. We're all looking for meaning and happiness. Perhaps self-tracking can help with one or more of those goals. Buster Benson has experimented enough over the years to at least give us some pointers.

Benson is the only subject of this book I'd met previously. That meeting was in January 2006 in Seattle, his hometown. I was on one of my regular trips to the US as a tech blogger and had come to Seattle for a Microsoft conference. I'd been communicating online with Erik Benson (as he was called back then) since 2003, and so I was looking forward to putting a face to the name. Previously employed by Seattle's other big computing company, Amazon.com, by early 2006 the 29-year-old Benson was building his own startup—a goal-tracking social network called "43Things." When I met him I got the impression that he was settled and content in the small, hip startup community of Seattle. But change, as always, was just around the corner for Erik Benson.

We kept in contact virtually, but it wasn't until seven years later that I next caught up with Benson in person. This time it wasn't in Seattle, but the headquarters of his new employer in San Francisco, Twitter. It was now January 2013 and since I'd last seen him, Benson had changed names twice, developed a string of social software products, run an art gallery in downtown Seattle, married for the second time and had a son. He'd done a lot over those seven years. But now with a young family to support, he had decided to return to the comfort of a full-time job. For all his changes over the years, it seemed like he was coming full circle. As with Amazon.com a decade before, Twitter was a cutting-edge—yet comfortable—environment for Benson to do what he does best: create change.

Twitter HQ is situated in a 1930s art deco building in San Francisco. The location is right on the border of the fashionable part of Market Street, where the seven-story Westfield Mall is, and the more downmarket part of Market Street populated by pawn shops, laundromats, and the type of run-down hotel that advertises itself in TripAdvisor as "near Union Square."

Although the Twitter building dates from an era well past, when I got off the elevator on the 6th floor I was surprised by the hip, modern decor of a Bay Area Internet company. A large, two-part lime-green sofa was the primary source of color in a spacious, brown-toned reception area. Set before the two sections of the sofa were two dark brown wooden coffee tables, each one artfully etched to look like a log. In front of the windows looking out to Market Street was a long, backlit glass reception desk, painted with wispy branch patterns and decorated with jagged faux-wood panels. Continuing the nature theme, the meeting rooms adjoining the reception area were all named after birds.

After I'd checked in at reception, I looked around for the fridge that is always present in any Internet company, big or small. Sure enough, Twitter had one directly across from the long desk. It was a large fridge with a glass door, well stocked with nutritious drinks. Knowing the protocol that the drinks are free at Internet companies, I helped myself to a low-sugar vitamin drink and sat down on the lime-green sofa to wait.

Buster Benson soon walked out to Twitter's reception area and greeted me. He's tall and lean, with tousled dark brown hair and a short scruffy beard. Today he was dressed in a smart-casual checkered brown shirt and blue jeans. His face is friendly, but reserved and always a bit anxious looking. When he smiles, which he does often, his smile is sometimes accompanied by a nervous chuckle. The overall impression I got from Benson was the same as seven years ago, when I first met him: he's a good-looking, hip guy, but there's something quiet and introspective about him. He looks as if he has a lot on his mind. Today it could have been a project he was working on at Twitter, the still recent move from Seattle to San Francisco for him and his family, his current self-tracking experiments, or a combination of those things and more. After an all too brief tour of Twitter HQ—there was a conference on that day, so it was busier than usual—we exited the building and walked to a local café to talk.

Portrait of the self-tracker as a young man

For as long as he can remember, Buster Benson has liked a challenge. His fascination with self-tracking started with personal challenges as a schoolboy, which he called "willpower experiments," along with an early habit of keeping journals. The challenges were sometimes of a social nature. In high school and college, he would organize and take part in challenges with his classmates. He described one example: "Everybody had to come up with a project and whoever didn't complete the project had to pay the other people $100." These youthful games got Buster Benson started in the world of self-tracking.

Challenging himself also led to his first full-time job. After graduating from college in 1998, he bet someone that he could get a job at Amazon.com—the then upstart Seattle e-commerce company. He won that bet, after learning HTML over a summer vacation and applying to Amazon.com as soon as he got back to Seattle. After a few years at the company and various side projects, including writing a self-published novel called *Man Versus Himself*, Benson began developing online self-tracking projects in 2003.

This was a period of experimentation on the Web. Nobody knew what the next big thing on the Internet would be after the dot com implosion of 2001. But there was a sense of adventure in the air. Developers and entrepreneurs of that time were thinking and tinkering. In mid-2003, for example, a Silicon Valley engineer named Mike Lee was mulling over an idea that would later turn into MyFitnessPal, an online calorie counter (we'll meet Mike in an upcoming chapter). In 2003 I was conducting my own little experiment when I started a technology blog called Read/Write Web in April of that year. I remember this period with fondness because we were all amateurs back then—trying things out on the Web, challenging ourselves to create change.

One of Erik Benson's early online self-tracking projects was called Mecember, which he started in December 2003. Unlike his current fairly simple and minimalist projects, Mecember was abstract and hard to understand. He described it at the time, grandly, as swapping places temporarily with "a Me in another dimension." But if you looked past the youthful philosophizing, essentially it came down to this: Benson would make simple changes to his lifestyle and track them, changes such as losing weight, or drinking less coffee. He wanted to note the daily effects on his body and mind of making those lifestyle changes. Reflecting on the project nine years later, Benson told me that despite achieving only mixed results, Mecember did teach him "on a very deep level that the more I understand the link between what I eat, drink, do … and how I feel, how healthy I am … the better."

Another of Benson's health-tracking projects was the "Morale-O-Meter," which he started in 2005. This was a long-running experiment that required him to rate his morale, every day, on a scale of 1–10. Again, the idea was to see how the things he did every day correlated to his daily health and how he felt. It was more than that though. The Morale-O-Meter was the first project in which Benson attempted to calculate his happiness, using his "morale" as a proxy. The Morale-O-Meter involved Benson counting things like the number of alcoholic and caffeinated drinks he had each day, number of hours of sleep, and his general health (which he rated 1–10 every day, with 10 being healthiest). He was hoping to discover that his morale score would, over time, closely correlate to his daily habits and health, which, he reasoned, would make it a good formula for happiness. Unfortunately, the Morale-O-Meter didn't provide him with the answers he was searching for. "After doing this for about three years," wrote Benson in a February 2009 blog post, "except for minor correlations between number of alcoholic drinks and amount of sleep, there were no deep insights."

A more successful Buster Benson project for making the connection between inputs (eating, drinking, personal actions) and outputs (feelings, health) was Health Month, which he launched in August 2010. It was a social network that enabled users to commit to a set of health-related challenges over the course of a calendar month, for example: "lose 5 pounds" or "limit drinking to 3 times per week." The idea was to update your progress every day and share it with other participants. The site attracted hundreds of users, including this author for a time. Happily for Benson, adding a social element to self-tracking turned out to be the missing link. It brought a sense of motivation to Benson's own self-tracking, with other participants cheering him on, and him doing the same for them. There was also a certain pride in achieving a health goal with one's peers looking on.

Anyone who rates themselves between one and ten every day for morale for over three years must be a compulsive personality. Buster Benson would agree with that, but he's careful to alleviate his obsessive streak by making his tracking projects fun. With Health Month, he took the fun quotient up a notch or two by introducing gaming elements into self-tracking. A term called "gamification" was all the rage in Silicon Valley at the time, meaning to add game-like features into a Web service—things like giving users badges and other virtual rewards such as tokens that could be used to buy things within an app.

Gamification became enormously popular over this period, 2009–2011, thanks to apps like Foursquare (a location check-in app, which awarded you the title of "mayor" if you checked in to a place more than anyone else) and FarmVille (a hokey Facebook game about virtual farming, as hugely annoying as it was hugely popular). Gamification elements motivated people to keep using these apps, despite having no monetary value and often being merely gimmicks. However, Buster Benson thought that gamification could provide real value in Health Month. So, to help motivate people to stick to their health goals, he introduced features such as a virtual Spin Wheel (to add an element of chance every day) and "Life points" to track your progress ("You start with 10, and lose 1 each time you break one of your rules").

Health Month was a leap forward for Benson in his self-tracking theories, but it wasn't a financial success. After losing $250,000 of angel investment on the venture, he sold the site in July 2012 to a two-man Canadian firm. Candidly, he wrote in a blog post at that time: "The last couple years have taught me that my life's creative purpose comes in the form of a question: 'How do we change ourselves?' All of my guesses so far have been mostly wrong."

Metamorphosis

By the time 2013 rolled around, Buster Benson was ready for a change of scene and a new challenge. Moving to San Francisco to take up a job with Twitter accomplished that. But at the same time he was determined to continue his self-tracking experiments. As we chatted in a café a couple of doors down from Twitter HQ, in late January 2013, I asked him what his current self-tracking project was. He told me it derived from a New Year's resolution. On January 1, 2013 he'd published to the Internet the following resolution: "At least 5 days a week, start my day proactively by doing at least one of these 6 things before looking at my phone: drink a glass of water, stretch, do pushups, do lunges, do plank, review my haiku deck."

Benson explained that his goal was to be more proactive first thing in the morning, to counteract his usual habit of "reactive responses" throughout the day. Doing one of the six activities would, he reasoned, give him positive momentum for the day. "I am very unmotivated to do anything in the morning," he admitted with a nervous laugh. "But I suspect that starting my day correctly will have an impact." Maybe it would even lead to less reactive responses later in the day. Ultimately, he's hoping to find out whether developing a morning habit will make him happier. That raises the possibility that even if he succeeds in becoming more proactive, he may conclude that he was happier being lazy first thing in the morning! He'd be back where he started. But this doesn't concern Benson, because all of his adult life has been an ongoing experiment. If this one doesn't work, he'll simply set himself a new challenge.

One of the keys to habit-forming is to make a conscious effort to do it regularly, until it becomes ingrained. But as everyone knows, it's easy to make a resolution. It's much harder to stick to it day in, day out. Benson, who now describes himself as an "amateur behavior change fanatic," admitted that he has the same problem that everyone else does: consistency. When we spoke he was nearly a month into his New Year's resolution, but he had already "fallen off the wagon." The life changes happening around him—the new job, moving his family from Seattle to San Francisco, a new apartment—made it difficult for him to stick to his resolution. "It definitely does not feel, yet, very easy," he admitted. "It's like torture almost! But if I can prove that it does make my day better, then that would be motivation to keep doing it."

The magic ingredient for meaningful change is motivation.

Having learned from Health Month that it's easier and more fun to stick to self-tracking goals if you make them social, Benson created a lightweight social network based on his resolution. Rather than develop a brand-new website, this time he chose to use an online mailing list: Google Groups. He started a group there and playfully named it the "Rabbit Rabbit Resolution Accountability Squad." The group encourages others to make a single resolution for the year, just as he did. At the beginning of each month, participants are to check in and report on their progress.

Despite his avid use of technology, Buster Benson is surprisingly skeptical of the current wave of consumer health products. While he's impressed with the design of health tracking devices like the Fitbit and Nike+ FuelBand wristband, he believes that the magic ingredient for meaningful change is often missing when people use these tools. That missing ingredient is, he believes, motivation.

"There are a lot of companies trying to create tools and services that help people change their behavior, improve their health, change their habits," Benson told me. But he thinks they rely on "a smokescreen of facts and studies" to push change. As an example, he cited faddish diets that claim that if you stick to them for 21 days, you've successfully developed a new eating habit. But these are "short-term marketing gimmicks," according to him. "There's an illusion of making your life better, but there's no long-term change happening." In Benson's view, the closest any organization has come to eliciting long-term change in people using these marketing techniques are the likes of Weight Watchers and Alcoholics Anonymous. However, he said, those organizations are not using new technologies; rather they rely on old-fashioned groups and "social support" strategies.

So how then can people improve their health and change their lifestyle habits? For Buster Benson, it comes down to a person's motivation. And that, he says, can't come from external sources. It has to come from within a person. "What causes a change," he explained, "is something you can't buy. It's something you have to have." He admitted that he doesn't know the answers to what best enables long-term change— that's why he experiments a lot with different self-tracking projects. But the path he's currently exploring is identity and belief change. "The idea that we cannot change our behaviors unless we change who we are," he said, "and who we think of ourselves as."

Benson used an example of a man who stands on a scale and sees that he weighs 200 pounds. "That disappoints him," he continued, "because he believes he's a lighter man than that. So he says to himself, 'I'm not that person. I'm actually a person who weighs 175 pounds.' That man is going to succeed at losing weight. His identity is as a 175-pound person, so he will do whatever it takes to get back to his reality of who he is and who he believes himself to be." Benson thinks this is why people are more likely to be successful at being a vegan, or vegetarian, or even a long-term runner. "They maintain habits for a long period of time because the label is an identity, it's not a behavior."

So the key to behavior change, according to Buster Benson's current theory, is understanding who you believe yourself to be, and whether or not you are that person right now. "And if you aren't," he added, "then any tool is going to help you, because you've already got the motivation." So, I asked, what if you believe you're a person who weighs 200 pounds, but you just don't like yourself being that weight? "Then it's a lot harder to do anything," he admitted.

Experimenting with his own identity has been a consistent theme in Buster Benson's self-tracking. We all do it, of course, typically in our youth, when we try on different personalities and poses to see what fits. Benson has pushed that type of experimentation a bit further, by changing his name twice. The first identity change occurred in September 2006 when he changed his name from Erik Benson to "Buster Butterfield McLeod." At the time he only meant to change his name for one year, as an art project. He claims to have done it "for no reason, as a sort of identity vacation" and that he wanted to see how it would affect his life "legally, socially and personally." The new surname, McLeod, was decided on a coin toss: "Heads for McLeod, tails for Butterfield." It landed heads. He was going to toss a coin again to select his first name, but wisely decided to choose "Buster." The alternatives were "Muppet" and "Benny"!

Behind the whimsical reason for the name change lay a series of upheavals in Benson's life during that time. In 2004, he had gotten divorced from his first wife, quit his job at Amazon and co-founded a startup. Going from a married man with a day job at a respectable company to a twenty-something single guy running a startup must have made him feel like a new person. Even so, most of us wouldn't have made such a drastic identity change. Even Benson himself didn't anticipate some of the problems he would encounter when he changed his name. He had to get a new social security card, driver's license, passport, library card, and much more. So the first thing the born-again Buster had to deal with was a lot of bureaucratic red tape.

Despite the initial hassle, the identity change proved to be a successful one for Buster McLeod. It led to a rejuvenation of his life and career, including fun experiments, such as founding a Seattle art gallery and bar called McLeod Residence. Indeed,

Buster had so much fun with his new self that he changed his own rules and kept the name, even after the one-year art project finished. In a blog post, he explained: "At first, I said that I would change it back. That was before I started a company with the name. Now it would be a little weird to go back. That said, I would like to eventually bring my old name back into the fold … perhaps as middle names." In October 2008 he changed his surname back to Benson after getting married for the second time. But, in a nod to his renewed self, he decided to keep the first name Buster.

Buster Benson's metamorphoses show that sometimes it's a long road to finding your true identity. Yet even though he's now happy with who he is, Benson is still looking for those elusive life insights.

Searching for epiphanies

Buster Benson is a self-described obsessive self-tracker on a quest for happiness. But he will often only track something about himself for a short period of time. In 2009 he wrote that the aim of self-tracking is to search for "epiphanies about yourself, about the cause and effect of things, in such a way that these numbers would eventually be able to tell you things about yourself that you didn't already know." In a sense, he's like a scientist—he'll gather some data about himself and come to an empirical conclusion based on that data. Once he's discovered something about himself that he didn't already know, he usually stops tracking it. Or the experiment simply fails. Sometimes the epiphanies haven't come, as Benson's various successes and failures over the years show. To see the scale of what Buster Benson tracks about himself, you only need to visit his website, busterbenson.com.

The website is crammed with data points and graphs about Benson's daily activities and emotions. It's unclear what the point of some of this tracking is, but you get the sense that Benson would rather over-track than under-track. At least he'll have a lot of data to use in future. Current things he's tracking about himself include how he's feeling at any one time, how many emails he gets and sends every day, where he's been, and even how many things he's posted to the Internet. One of his more playful tracking projects is to document what he's doing every Tuesday at 7 p.m. As at the time of writing, the top activities at 7 p.m. every Tuesday for Buster Benson are: having dinner (34% of the time), drinking (13%), and traveling (9%).

Many of the things Benson tracks are relatively unimportant—even trivial. But not all of it is. "I track meaningful one-on-one time with my family," Benson told me, adding that he is certain it correlates to his happiness. "By tracking it, I remember that I know this has an impact." In other words, he tracks quality time with his family as a constant reminder of what's really important in life. So self-tracking needn't be a selfish thing. Indeed, tracking has always been about much more than himself for Buster Benson. He's not just aiming to improve his own lifestyle, but those of the people who share it with him. Perhaps a big reason for that is due to the passing of his own father, who died when Benson was only seventeen.

You might think that an avid quantified-self proponent like Benson would be a highly logical person, since he defines himself by data. To use a popular culture reference, if any character from Star Trek was a self-tracker, it would surely be Dr. Spock and not Captain Kirk. But one of the surprising things about Benson is that he's a mix of the structured and unstructured. He's half Spock, half Kirk. Benson told me that he hates to be controlled—even by himself. That's very Kirk-like. Yet he is also rigorous about implementing rules for his life. Very Spock-like. To strike a balance between logical and happy-go-lucky, some of Benson's rules call for random or unpredictable behavior. For example: he changed his name, yet used a coin toss to determine the final outcome.

What Buster Benson is doing with his self-imposed rules is not unusual. Many an artist, writer, and musician has enhanced their creativity by imposing rules on themselves in order to create within a framework. One of the most popular bands in the 2000s, the White Stripes, created a vivid artistic world from a few constrictive rules. The band, composed of singer-guitarist Jack White and drummer Meg White, dressed only in three colors (red, white, and black). All their album covers and videos used that restricted palette. It wasn't just the color scheme; the music itself had rules. The song structure, according to White, revolved around three things (storytelling, melody, and rhythm) and the band relied on only three instruments (guitar, drums, and vocals). Such constriction was a means to "force ourselves to create," explained Jack White in a documentary. The point is that Jack White likes rules, at least those he imposes on himself. So does Buster Benson. For both men, the self-imposed rules create a framework. For White, the framework is how he creates music. For Benson, the framework is how he lives his life.

The other benefit of self-imposed rules is that they make you think about what you're doing. The musician Brian Eno's whole career has been built on a foundation of rules and constrictions. One of the founding members of 1970s band Roxy Music, and a highly regarded solo artist and producer since the mid-70s, Eno used to record entire albums based on a deck of instruction cards, each with a random aphorism on it like "Only one element of each kind" or "Work at a different speed." In a 2010 BBC radio interview with Eno, singer and part-time DJ Jarvis Cocker commented that Eno's strategies "stop people being on auto-pilot." In a similar way, Buster Benson's self-tracking experiments often prod him to do something that gets him out of a rut or routine—for example, his morning resolution to do one of six activities before he looks at his iPhone.

However, you should never let the rules control you. The way Buster Benson tries to avoid that is to de-emphasize numbers in tracking. In a presentation in December 2012, entitled "Why I self-track," Benson noted that "precision can be counter-productive." So instead of tracking the number of steps he does a day, for Benson it's sufficient to note that he "walked to work." Instead of counting calories in his lunch, he prefers to simply register that he "ate a salad." Instead of tracking how many hours in a day he works, Benson tracks whether he "did meaningful work." In all of these cases, Benson is rejecting numbers and instead uses subjective criteria. It's his way of not getting too obsessed with data.

What about objective things about the body, such as DNA? It turns out that Buster Benson has a big interest in his genome too, although he thinks it's "meaningless data right now." He predicts it won't become truly useful for another ten or so years. Having said that, Benson told me that one of his first interests as a kid was genetics. He wanted to be a genetic biologist: "I wanted to invent animals … turns out the technology's not there yet." Nevertheless, on April 11, 2011, Benson signed himself, his wife Kellianne, and one-year-old son Niko up for a DNA test at consumer genetics company 23andMe. In a brave move, even for someone who had already published a lot of personal data about himself on the Web, Benson decided to make his genome data public. Although, in typical fashion, it turned out that this decision was motivated by a challenge he'd set himself for 2011: "My motto for the year is 'talk it out.' Step one is to try to push the boundaries about what I'm willing to be public about."

Curiously, posting his life code (DNA) motivated him to also publish a set of highly subjective documents: "My beliefs, my life list, my yearly birthday mottos, my manifesto for extraordinary living." He adds to each of these documents from time to time and the software he uses keeps a copy of each version. His aim is to "track changes" in the data set over time and "treat my sense of self as a codebase." Perhaps one day in the future, he posits, he or someone else will be able to correlate his beliefs and life list with his genetic data.

As you can see, Buster Benson is really pushing the boundaries of self-tracking. He's almost trying to program himself, like a computer. Indeed, most of his self-tracking is Boolean, just like a software programing language. In other words, his tracking inputs are often true or false, with logical if/then conclusions. If it's true that Benson walked to work today, then therefore he is happy (for the "walking" part of his self-programing at least). He even has a formula for calculating his daily happiness, which is a series of eight true/false questions that he asks himself at the end of each day.

Each question (for example: Did I spend quality time with my son?) gets one point if answered "true" for that day. The higher the points tally each day, the happier he is … until the Kirk in him objects to that logic!

True or false: is Buster happy?

It's difficult to judge how another person truly feels about him or herself. However, my sense is that Buster Benson is a relatively happy man when it comes down to it, particularly since his second marriage and the birth of his son. But only he knows for sure—a formula won't give us the answer. There's a limit to how far Benson can take the computing analogy. He's only human after all, and sometimes life cannot be distilled into easily tracked bits.

As we wound down our interview, I asked Benson if he will always track things about himself. "I hope so," he replied, with his familiar nervous chuckle. I believe it, because what really drives Buster Benson is a perpetual restlessness. He will always be trying to improve aspects of himself. He will continue to change things about himself and develop new habits. This year it's trying to be more proactive, next year it will be something else.

I myself will never do as much self-tracking as Buster Benson—and I don't advise it for others either. But we can learn from his ongoing experiments. He's shown us that you don't necessarily need to track

> **What drives Buster Benson is a perpetual restlessness. He will always be trying to improve himself.**

something for a long time for it to provide useful—and usable—data. On the other hand, for things of great importance, like meaningful time with one's family, self-tracking can be a good way to stay mindful about your daily activities.

Buster Benson's obsessive self-tracking is primarily about improving himself and finding happiness. However, it's also leaving a digital trail of his daily existence—what he did every day, what he felt, what he's trying to change about himself at any one time, what he believes in. In his beliefs file, Benson states that he is essentially agnostic. "Souls don't exist separate from the physical body," he declares. However, he does believe in the Singularity (the notional moment when computers outstrip human intelligence). If we accept his beliefs, then in 100 years Buster Benson's identity will only exist in digital form—the daily self-tracking notes he published on the Internet, the software he created over his life, the self-tracking numbers and Boolean digits he recorded every day of his adult existence. Yet strangely, for someone so intent on recording his daily life online, Benson's previous home page—erikbenson.com—has already slipped into the hands of a domain spammer. He let the domain name expire. Ironically, erikbenson.com now re-directs to TrafficForJesus.com.

In the final analysis, I suspect it doesn't worry Buster Benson too much whether his digital legacy survives 100 years from now. Because if Darwin obliges, he will continue to live on through his son and any other descendants he may have. I'm pretty sure that very human notion, which can't be tracked in his own lifetime, satisfies Buster Benson.

CHAPTER TWO

THE PEDOMETER ON STEROIDS: TRACKING ACTIVITY WITH FITBIT

The trend in these devices has been: how do they become more integrated into people's lifestyles?

Eric Friedman, co-founder of Fitbit

It was a fine winter's day in San Francisco's sprawling Golden Gate Park, sometime in early 2007. The morning mist had tapered off, giving passing joggers a clear view of an awkward-looking cycling and running duo. One was a tall, bespectacled European man, named Eric Friedman, who was riding a bicycle in that gangly way tall men have. Running directly behind him was a shorter Asian man called James Park. What was odd about the pair was that they were connected by a series of cords. On the back of Friedman's bike was a portable electronics board from which the cords sprouted. At the other end of the wires was Park, who was trying to jog at a steady pace. It was Friedman's job not to disrupt Park's running rhythm, which meant not going too fast on the bike. But the bulky electronics panel was making that difficult. So the bike swerved involuntarily every minute or so as Friedman struggled to maintain control. As the pair passed bemused joggers and people walking their dogs, Friedman grimly cycled on—every now and then nervously looking back to check on the gap between his bike and the puffing James Park.

The point of all this was to capture information from Park's body via sensors that were attached to his chest, arms, and legs. That data was transmitted into the electronics board through the cords attached to the sensors. Afterwards, the pair studied the output. The key piece of data was how many steps James Park took while he was running. But they also wanted to cross-check that with motion data from other parts of the body, such as movement of the arms. The idea was to calculate not just steps, but the intensity of the workout, from which they would then figure out the calorie burn. Friedman and Park were making their first steps toward building a new kind of pedometer, one that was both more accurate and more useful than traditional step-counting devices.

It took more than two years to get from the Golden Gate Park data collection experiments to an actual product, called the "Fitbit Tracker." Far removed from the bulky electronics board that Eric Friedman had carried on his bicycle two years earlier, the Fitbit Tracker was a tiny device that you clipped onto your belt. At first glance, it looked like a miniature version of the monolith in the movie *2001: A Space Odyssey*. It was rectangular, sleekly dark, and smooth all over. But if you looked closer, it had a single button on it, which when pressed showed various bits of information about your activity: how many steps you'd taken, distance traveled, calories consumed, and amount of sleep.

Friedman and Park had succeeded in creating a next-generation pedometer. They called it a pedometer on steroids.

Starting a long journey

The Fitbit office of today is located in the heart of San Francisco's financial district, where tall buildings obscure the sun and ensconce the area in shadow. It was a fine but cold winter's day in January 2013 when I made my way to the office to meet Eric Friedman. While the outside was dominated by bland skyscrapers, inside the Fitbit office it was a welcoming raft of bright green and red, set in iPod-white surroundings.

While I was admiring the interior, Eric Friedman came out

to the foyer to meet me. He's tall and lean, with neat brown hair and oval-shaped engineer's glasses. On this day, he was dressed tidily in an orange-checked long-sleeved shirt and tan slacks. His carefully color-coordinated attire nicely complemented the modern Apple Computer-inspired office decor. As we sat down to talk, Friedman fixed his eyes on me attentively and politely. With that earnest, quiet, sing-song voice that many Silicon Valley computer scientists possess, Friedman explained to me how he and James Park came up with the idea for Fitbit. "When we started thinking about what to do next," he said, "something in the consumer space was always a primary focus for us. We talked about GPS and other kinds of sensor technology." Friedman paused and smiled. "Then the Nintendo Wii came out."

The Nintendo Wii was launched in November 2006 and its handheld remote controller was an immediate sensation in the gaming world. Traditional gaming controllers, from the likes of Sony PlayStation and Microsoft Xbox, were operated by wiggling a joystick and pressing buttons. But the Wii Remote was a game changer.

It was operated by simply waving the controller around in the air. This was achieved through motion-sensing technology that allowed Wii games to be controlled by gestures and pointing. For Friedman and Park, the Wii Remote was a revelation—it showed them the possibilities of motion sensors. With their background in the Internet world, the pair began to think of possible applications for motion sensing in other consumer products.

The primary technology inside the Wii was a sensor called an accelerometer, which senses motion. It was to become the linchpin of the Fitbit device too. Initially Friedman and Park were thinking of a wearable sensor device that could be used for personalized coaching in sports, but this idea soon morphed into a much broader one. The challenge, explained Friedman, was: "How do we do all-day wear in a fun and personable way?" Whereas the Wii was a gaming machine, designed for relatively short and sporadic usage, Friedman and Park were thinking about something a person might wear most of the day and night. "For us," Friedman continued, "all-day wear included where you go for your walk, your run, how you sleep—all that stuff. But how do we track that and how do we then make that data fun, interesting and, most importantly, actionable?"

This line of thought led to the Golden Gate Park experiments at the beginning of 2007. By May 2007, Friedman and Park had settled on the idea they would pursue: a new type of step-counter (aka pedometer) that would connect to the Internet. They created a new company to begin work on this idea, named Fitbit.

Friedman and Park were no strangers to startup life. Fitbit was the pair's third startup together and they'd already experienced the success of an acquisition. Their second startup, a photo-sharing website called Webshots, was sold to media company CNET in 2005. By May 2007, the pair had completed their two-year earnout with CNET (the amount of time they were contractually obliged to work for their acquirer). There was no question they would collaborate again on another startup, since both enjoyed creating new products and they complemented each other perfectly. It was a Silicon Valley dream team, the kind of partnership that venture capitalists drool over: a super-smart engineer partnered with a savvy CEO. Eric Friedman was the software brains, with his computer science degree from Yale and intense engineer's mind. James Park was the more extroverted personality, who thrived on sales and marketing challenges.

A pedometer is a device that measures steps and distances in walking or running. Traditionally, pedometers have used a mechanical switch to detect steps, along with a simple counter. The modern way to measure steps is to use an accelerometer. As the name suggests, this little sensor measures the acceleration of your body—in other words, whenever your body moves. The Fitbit Tracker's accelerometer enables it to sense periodic motion consistent with walking. Fitbit will also estimate your stride length, based on the height and weight figures you input into its website when you first start using the device. These were just some of the things that Eric Friedman and James

Park were testing with their cycling and running double act at Golden Gate Park.

Capturing accurate step data from a very small pedometer device was the first big challenge for the pair. The device needed to differentiate walking from, for example, riding a scooter across a bumpy road. This was more difficult than they first imagined. "Turns out, older people have slightly irregular gaits," said Friedman, "which looks a lot like riding a bus on a bumpy street." The Fitbit Tracker would have to be able to tell the difference. "How do you identify people's gaits when they're older, ill, or injured?" Even now, telling me of this research conundrum from six years ago, Eric Friedman wore a look of mock exasperation. But there were even trickier design issues to overcome: how would people carry the Fitbit device, and how would that affect measurement? "What if you want to stick it in your pocket?" said Friedman, his bespectacled eyes widening in a mixture of engineering delight and horror. "And what if it's sitting there rotating in your pocket?" He adjusted his glasses and leaned forward. "Well, then you can't use gravity—and that completely breaks all those physics models." He leaned back again, adding that battery power was yet another design obstacle. How would they create a small pedometer device that did all this whizzy stuff, but didn't need charging every day?

Once Friedman and Park had finally overcome the data collection issues, they turned their attention to figuring out how best to present the data to the user. Friedman set to work developing algorithms to convert the raw data from the accelerometer into useful information about activity—things like steps walked, calories burned, and distance traveled. James Park explained in a January 2009 blog post how Fitbit developed its algorithms. "Our approach is that we have test subjects wear the Fitbit while also wearing a device that produces a 'truth value'," he wrote. For example, to develop the algorithms for step counting, Fitbit had test subjects wear the prototype Fitbit device while also carrying a click counter and clicking off steps. This process took up a good portion of the 2007 and 2008 period, because the algorithms required a lot of experimentation and test data. "Sometimes the algorithms you develop work very well in one case but completely fail in another," explained Park.

Another challenge for Friedman and Park was the user interface—specifically, how to present various pieces of information to users on such a small device. They wanted it to be more than just the number of steps, but there was only room for one thing to display at a time. The solution was to add a small button onto the mini monolith, allowing users to click through the different numbers—steps, calories, distance, and more. The pair also put a lot of thought into how to make that data more appealing. As Eric Friedman explained to me: "We really struggled with how numbers are boring, compared to graphical information." What the pair came up with was a pretty icon of a flower on the Tracker screen. At the start of the day, you'd see just the bottom of the flower. But as you went through your day and got closer to your daily steps goal, the rest of the flower would be sketched in. Once you reached your goal, the whole flower would display. It was a simple yet effective way of enabling users to track their progress over the day without flashing numbers at them.

During this initial design period over 2007 and 2008, Friedman and Park began to think about what form their pedometer device would take. They commissioned a top industrial design firm, New Deal Design, to come up with ideas. The design concepts considered included a small circular device to be carried in a mini holster on the user's belt, a square clip-on, a square "solid block" that the user would put in their pocket or purse, an oval-shaped "loop" that could be tied to a necklace or belt, and a wristband (the concept that Fitbit's competitors Nike and Jawbone eventually went with). But one design concept from New Deal Design stood out for Friedman and Park: a small rectangular belt clip-on. The design firm, wary that its clients were Silicon Valley geeks, likened this winning concept to "a thumb-drive for fitness."

Fitbit's engineering team went to work on a prototype, but soon got their first taste of the manufacturing problems that would plague the startup over the next couple of years. The first prototype turned out to be noticeably thicker than the design concept. In a January 2009 blog post, James Park explained that this was because "it was very difficult to fit all the components into the shape." However, the pair pressed forward. They wanted to debut the prototype device at the September 2008 TechCrunch 50 conference in San Francisco. TechCrunch 50 was an event at which 50 startups presented their fledgling products to expert panelists—like an *American Idol* for startups.

When James Park presented the "Fitbit Tracker" prototype to this audience of Silicon Valley geeks and fellow entrepreneurs in September 2008, the expectation was that it would be available for purchase before the end of that year, for $99. That was just a few months away. However, it took more than twelve months for the first Fitbit devices to finally ship.

Climbing the manufacturing mountain

Eric Friedman has always enjoyed climbing hills. "If there's something to climb, I've gotta climb it," he told me in his earnest manner. When he was school age, Friedman did cross-country running and competitive biking. I can easily imagine his tall, gangly frame running briskly across a park in Pittsburgh, where he grew up. At the time he owned a GPS watch and sporadically tracked these activities, primarily by writing his statistics down in a journal. "But I often got lazy and stopped," he told me. The manual effort involved in tracking his runs wasn't something he could sustain, like many of us who begin to track something and find that it's too much trouble. That was one of the motivating forces behind the Fitbit Tracker—it was something you'd wear every day and it would automatically track your activity and wirelessly log it on the Fitbit website. In his mid-thirties now, Friedman is married and has a young son. These days his main activity is going for walks with his wife—although he still likes the challenge of a good hill.

If Eric Friedman and his business partner James Park expected to easily climb the hill of hardware manufacturing in a couple of months, they soon discovered it was a mountain.

It took a whole year to climb. Soon after TechCrunch50 in September 2008, Fitbit opened up its website for pre-orders. The intention was to take advantage of the upcoming holidays. But when Christmas passed and the New Year began with no Fitbit Trackers in sight, people who had pre-ordered the device began to ask questions. On the Fitbit blog in late January 2009, co-founder and CEO Park expressed his frustration at the delays. "When we launched at TechCrunch," he wrote in a comment responding to an impatient customer, "we expected the Dec[ember] launch date and we had major PR events scheduled for the holiday season that we eventually had to pull out of."

That included missing the prestigious Consumer Electronics Show (CES) in Las Vegas in early January 2009, the biggest consumer gadget event of the year. Fitbit had already been named top gadget in the Health and Wellness category at CES, so to not show up at the event was an embarrassment to the young startup. Park blamed "the slippage" on "being ultraconservative with product reliability and the fact that each design tweak takes at least one to two weeks to prototype and verify." In fact, Fitbit had underestimated the complexity of producing its mini monolith in mass quantities. This was Friedman and Park's first hardware company and with over 100 electronic components plus 22 plastic and metal parts inside its small rectangular casing, the Fitbit Tracker was a complex gadget. Park told the *New York Times* that it took them eight months just to refine its prototype into something that was ready to manufacture. There were further delays in the testing phase, including equipment getting stuck in customs in Indonesia.

> **With over 100 electronic components plus 22 plastic and metal parts, the Fitbit Tracker was a complex gadget.**

The problems stemmed from the pair's desire to sell the Fitbit device at under $100 so that it would fit any budget. Friedman and Park made an early decision to take a low-cost approach. According to James Park in a November 2008 blog post, that meant "picking the most cost-effective components that can meet the requirements and also developing a mechanical design that is cheap to manufacture and assemble in high volumes." They also soon discovered that while some of the production could be automated (primarily the circuit board, the computing part of the device), a lot of the assembly of the Fitbit had to be done by hand. "In order to keep the manual labor costs low," continued Park's blog post, "we decided to assemble the Fitbit overseas in Singapore and Batam, Indonesia."

By December 2008 Friedman and Park were in Singapore watching "production prototypes" being built. This was the intermediate stage, between the initial design prototype that was shown off at TechCrunch 50 a few months earlier, and the final product. The idea with the production prototype was to "uncover any remaining issues and to tweak the design before the Fitbit is sent off to mass production." But even at this stage, the signs were worrying. James Park listed a number of problems with the production prototype: the 30-minute assembly time (far too long for mass production), the button was too stiff, the charging contact mechanism was "unreliable," and more.

In Park's January 2009 blog post, he complained that the charging problem had become "the bane of our existence." It would take another four months to get that fixed. In May 2009, Park wrote: "If you remember, we had charging reliability problems in our early prototypes and it took forever to get those contacts right." Sadly, it wasn't the end of the manufacturing issues. With more than a hint of exasperation, Park wrote about a new battery problem. "Our battery supplier delivered our batteries last week, but most of them were about 1 mm too long, which prevented them from fitting inside the Fitbit." He added, rather hopefully, "I actually just got word from them an hour ago that the new batch of batteries will be ready by June 4th, so this won't cause any delays." Another four months later, in September 2009, the product finally shipped—at least to the customers who had pre-ordered it twelve months before.

"Thanks everyone for your patience!" wrote an exhausted James Park.

Walking 10,000 steps a day

Despite the delays, Fitbit garnered good reviews when people started using it from September 2009 on. However, initially there was some skepticism about the actual health benefits of using a Fitbit Tracker. Eric Friedman admitted that even his own father—who he described as a "mad scientist type, hair all over the place"—pooh-poohed the device. But his dad, who has type 2 diabetes, changed his mind when he began to use the Fitbit Tracker to monitor his daily activity. Friedman senior was soon walking an average of 20,000 steps a day, which delighted his son. "Seeing him lose weight, seeing that change, was incredible," he remarked.

Eric Friedman learned things about his own body, too, when he was trialing the Fitbit Tracker. On testing early versions of the Fitbit Tracker, he was surprised at how few steps he took most days, as little as 800 steps in one day, if he worked from home and didn't leave his San Francisco apartment. He also discovered that the number of calories people use when doing exercise varies between people, sometimes significantly. Friedman's girlfriend at the time (and now wife) went on runs, but to his amazement she burned fewer calories than he did sitting in his apartment working.

As for me, I bought my first Fitbit Tracker in 2011 and wore it daily for a few months. Like Friedman, at first I was surprised at how few steps I took in a day. I shouldn't have been, since I write for a living and so I'm sitting at a computer most of my day. But still, having the raw numbers in front of you is surprisingly motivating in terms of keeping active every day. It also gives you a baseline, so you can begin to set yourself daily targets to improve your activity levels. This is a fairly common experience, according to Fitbit's statistics. James Park said at the 2013 CES conference that after using a Fitbit tracking device the average user is "about 40% more active after about 12 weeks." In other words, people become motivated to get more active after they start using the Fitbit pedometer.

To see how other Fitbit users are making use of the Fitbit Tracker, I browsed the message boards on Fitbit's website. It seems that most users just want to be more active every day and the Fitbit device provides them with the motivation to do that. "Now I'm constantly trying to find ways to add activity into my day," one message read. Setting yourself challenges is also popular. One Fitbit user said on the company's forums that she doubled her activity level "just to challenge myself and keep my numbers up."

In terms of specific goals that Fitbit users strive for, losing weight is of course very popular. For Donna Allen, a 65-year-old from Fountain Valley, California, this was her primary goal when she purchased a Fitbit in April 2012. "I've battled being overweight since I was a child," she told me via email. "I've always been fairly active, [but] not active enough." Her first goal was to reach the 10,000 steps per day that Fitbit recommends. "I'm very competitive," she said, "so that goal was reached within a month." She then joined some of the Fitbit groups (Active with Fitbit, Climb Every Mountain Co-Op, John Olsen Walk, and Appalachian Trail). All of those groups challenged her to walk and climb stairs, which helped her to lose weight. She also used a food tracking app to match up her calories expended by walking to calories consumed from eating. "I wasn't dieting, just making sure I expended at least 500 calories per day more than I ate," she commented. The result of all this Fitbit-inspired activity was that Donna Allen lost 50 pounds and went from a size 16 to size 4. She now regularly walks over 20,000 steps a day, mainly through jogging on a mini trampoline and walking her two poodles.

Twenty thousand steps per day is a lot! During my own experiments with the Fitbit Tracker, I settled for 8,000 steps per day as my daily goal, which for me requires a bit of effort each day to achieve since I work from home in a sedentary job. For example, I try to go for a daily walk to my local café, which takes me about ten or eleven minutes to reach. The Fitbit Tracker told me that walking to the café from my home office equals about 1,500 steps. So walking to and from my favorite café is 3,000 steps in total, depressingly only a third of my daily activity goal. Therefore to achieve my 8,000-step goal, I either need to go for another walk in the evening, or do something equally active (such as walk around a shopping mall).

As Donna noted, Fitbit itself recommends 10,000 steps per day—roughly equivalent to five miles (eight kilometers). Ten thousand is also the number of steps recommended by the American Heart Association to improve health and decrease the risk of heart disease. So it's a commonly accepted yardstick for an active lifestyle.

The origin of the 10,000 steps per day metric can be traced back to the 1960s, when a Japanese company called Yamasa Corporation created a pedometer with the nickname of "manpo-kei," which, literally translated, means "ten thousand steps meter." Japanese walking clubs began using the Yamasa device, and the 10,000-steps metric was further popularized by Dr. Yoshiro Hatano, a Japanese researcher at the Kyushu University of Health and Welfare. He came up with the slogan "10,000 steps per day for better health."

Since the 1960s, several academic studies have backed up the 10,000 figure. Ten thousand steps was defined as an "active" lifestyle by the President's Council on Fitness, Sports & Nutrition, in a study published in 2004. The paper also classified less than 5,000 steps per day as "sedentary," 5,000–7,499 as "low active" and "typical of daily activity excluding sports/exercise," 7,500–9,999 as "somewhat active," and more than 12,500 as "highly active." The report admitted, however, that the 10,000 steps per day goal for an "active" lifestyle may not be achievable for some groups, such as the elderly and people living with chronic illness. A 2008 report by the American College of Sports Medicine agreed with the classification in the President's Council report, but advocated separate guidelines for children aged six to twelve.

Although 10,000 steps per day is recommended by Fitbit for an "active" lifestyle—and as you can see there is solid scientific evidence that this number is a good recommendation—it may not be practical for you. It takes a concerted effort to get to 10,000 steps per day if you have a relatively sedentary job or lifestyle. Particularly enthusiastic walkers, or those with a lot of time on their hands, can get up to 20,000 steps per day. But most of us would struggle to reach half that every day.

It really comes down to one of the basic principles of self-tracking: test for yourself what works. Jenny Ruhl, author of the book *Diet 101* and one of my favorite nutrition experts, said this about monitoring the effects of a new diet: "You should test things and see what they do for you, not look to authorities." She was specifically referring to testing blood sugar levels, but the same principle applies to monitoring how many steps you do in a day.

Using the Fitbit over a period of time (it doesn't matter how long), find out what level of daily activity works for your body and your lifestyle. For me, I discovered that 8,000 steps per day is sufficient. That keeps my weight level and my body happy. But more importantly for my particular lifestyle, it pushes me to get off my computer a couple of times a day and do some walking, preferably outside, to my local café or the shops, so I get fresh air as well as exercise. That feels like an active enough lifestyle for my purposes.

"You should test things and see what they do for you, not look to authorities."

From the early days of riding a bike through Golden Gate Park, with step-tracking cords attached to his jogging co-founder James Park, to the current era of multiple Fitbit devices, I was curious to know how Eric Friedman himself uses Fitbit now. In the heart of San Francisco's business district, sitting in a modern office which includes a couple of treadmill desks, I asked Eric Friedman what value he gets from his Fitbit devices.

"So, I'm really interested in the trends," Eric Friedman told me in his quiet, sing-song voice. He also likes to track distance, especially "on days or weeks where I'm doing something out of this world." That's because "it's much harder to move the needle on distance." But like most Fitbit users, counting steps is what gives Eric Friedman the most value. Steps are useful to so many people because they're "so measurable," he remarked. He doesn't have any specific body-based goals, such as losing weight or improving his endurance. He simply wants to stay active every day and Fitbit helps him measure that.

At this point, Eric Friedman paused and considered for a moment—as if he had just initiated a software algorithm on his computer. "I would not have predicted this," he said, looking at me as if the results of his algorithm had just come in. "I thought it [Fitbit] was going to be very caloric-burn based, but I think that it's definitely steps for me. It's just really fun."

In other words, despite all of the sophistication packed into this small device and the fancy data streams, at its heart Fitbit is a step counter.

Tracing previous tracks

In fact the Fitbit Tracker is the latest in a long line of pedometer devices. Two very famous people from history are closely associated with the early development of the pedometer: the master Italian artist Leonardo da Vinci and the third president of the United States, Thomas Jefferson, although the history of step-counting goes back much further even than Leonardo. It was in fashion as far back as the second and third centuries AD, when the Roman Empire used steps to determine distances for its military maps.

In addition to painting masterpieces like the *Mona Lisa* in the late 15th and early 16th centuries, Leonardo da Vinci made many inventive sketches of possible future mechanical devices. He famously sketched flying machines, centuries before the first airplane was invented. It turns out he also sketched a very early version of a pedometer device. One of da Vinci's notebooks contains a sketch of a "pendulum," which looks kind of like a wheelbarrow. When pushed, the pendulum would move back and forth in correlation with the movements of the walker's body. According to Charles H. Gibbs-Smith, in his 1978 book, *The Inventions of Leonardo da Vinci*, da Vinci designed his pedometer to help create accurate maps. But like most of his sketched designs for mechanical devices, the pendulum was never built.

Thomas Jefferson was one of the Founding Fathers of

America and the principal author of the Declaration of Independence in 1776. He went on to become the third president, from 1801 to 1809. It's sometimes claimed that Jefferson invented the pedometer, but in fact he was more like an early adopter who helped popularize the device in the United States. On a visit to France in February 1786, Jefferson wrote to his friend and colleague James Madison, offering to purchase a watch for him. But he also added, "For 12 louis more you can have in the same cover, but on the back side & absolutely unconnected with the movements of the watch, a pedometer which shall render you an exact account of the distances you walk."

Another device Jefferson used was strapped between waist and knee in order to calculate the number of strides he made when walking. In a letter to J. Bannister, Junior, on June 19, 1787, Jefferson wrote: "Are you become a great walker? You know I preach up that kind of exercise. Shall I send you a conte-pas [a pedometer]? It will cost you a dozen louis, but be a great stimulus to walking, as it will record your steps."

Jefferson was an avid walker and a keen adopter of the latest technology. If he were alive today, you can bet he'd be logging all kinds of fitness data into Fitbit or a similar product! But in fact neither da Vinci nor Jefferson was responsible for the pedometer. If there is any one inventor, it was the Swiss watchmaker Abraham-Louis Perrelet. Perrelet's most famous invention was an automatic pocket watch, in 1770. The self-winding mechanism was, in effect, powered by a pedometer. In a report to the Geneva Society of Arts in 1776, H. B. de Saussure described the mechanism: "Master Perrelet, watchmaker, has made a watch in such a way that it winds itself in the wearer's pocket as he walks; fifteen minutes of walking suffices to make the watch run eight days." In 1780, ten years after the self-winding pocket watch, Perrelet created the first pedometer. It specifically measured steps and distance while walking.

The modern era of electronic pedometers began in the 1960s. Yamasa Corporation in Japan, where the 10,000 steps per day metric originated, produced some of the most accurate electronic pedometers of that era. Cheap pedometers have also been used over the years as marketing giveaways by massive consumer companies like Coca-Cola and McDonald's. In 2004 the burger chain McDonald's, a frequent target for healthy lifestyle proponents, tried to assuage its critics by giving away a plastic pedometer in a combo meal for adults. Called "The Go Active! Meal," the promotion included the plastic pedometer, a bottle of water, a salad, and an exercise booklet. Alas, the promotion can't have been very successful—it lasted barely a month.

Pedometers received a big boost in popularity when they began to be integrated into some of the most popular entertainment gadgets toward the end of the first decade of this century. Nintendo was once again an early mover. On November 1, 2008—just a month after Fitbit announced its product at TechCrunch50—Nintendo released a game for the Nintendo DS device entitled "Personal Trainer: Walking." The game included two pedometers, which connected to the game card via infrared signals. Soon after, Apple began to integrate pedometers into its iPod Nano product line. The fifth-generation iPod Nano product included a pedometer. That was announced in September 2009, about when Fitbit began to ship its first Trackers. A year later, in September 2010, the sixth-generation iPod Nano was released and it too included a pedometer.

As for Eric Friedman, he has a deep respect for the long history of pedometers. For his birthday a couple of years ago, his father gave him a collection of classic pedometers. The oldest is a pedometer from around 1880.

Stepping into the future

Fitbit is the latest generation of the pedometer, along with similar "Wearable Internet" devices such as the Nike FuelBand and Jawbone UP. Wearable Internet products will continue to evolve and any attempt to catalogue them in a book is doomed to be out of date before it's published. Fitbit alone has released several new versions of its Tracker since 2009, including in new forms (it finally released a wristband to compete with Nike and Jawbone in January 2013). Along the way Fitbit has added new features and streamlined the design of its Tracker. The second-generation device, the Fitbit Ultra, released in October 2011, added an altimeter to track how many floors you climb each day. It does this by measuring barometric pressure— in other words, changes in air pressure when you walk up or down. Also new in generation two were supportive messages ("Congratulations, you've reached your step goal for today!"), a clock, and stopwatch.

What Fitbit tracks will also evolve over time. From early on, it wasn't just steps. It also claimed to measure "sleep quality," by calculating how much you move in your bed. To do this, the Tracker is simply tucked into an armband at night. Some of Fitbit's competitors already track blood pressure and other body metrics, so it's a safe assumption that Fitbit will further extend what it tracks over the coming years.

Fitbit has branched out into other fitness-related products too. In January 2012 it released a WiFi-enabled scale called the Fitbit Aria. It was a very similar product to another WiFi scale that had become popular with self-tracking early adopters, the Withings WiFi Body Scale. The Withings scale was released in its home country, France, in June 2009 and in the US and Europe in September of that year (the same month that the original Fitbit Tracker went on sale). The Withings scale measures weight and body mass, automatically uploading the results to a companion website. The Fitbit Aria scale does the same thing and was a welcome addition to the Fitbit product range, because now users could correlate their daily activity to their daily weight.

So the Fitbit Tracker, as a clip-on device, is far from being the endgame in wearable technology. Indeed the Fitbit Tracker may well come to be seen, in time, as a product akin to the iPod at the start of this century. While the iPod was innovative in its day, it soon got usurped by the iPhone's ever-increasing storage capacity and ability to stream music from apps like Spotify. The Fitbit Tracker in 2013 is likewise one of the most prominent wearable technology products of its era, but it too may soon be made redundant. There are already startups experimenting with sensors woven into T-shirts, for example. If you have an accelerometer integrated into your clothes, why would you need to clip it on your belt? Sensors in your clothing isn't even a new concept. Sports shoe manufacturer Nike was one of the first companies to experiment in this area, with its Nike+ running shoe (with sensor technology) dating back to 2006.

In September 2014, Apple announced a new wearable product called the Apple Watch. It's the most sophisticated offering yet in the emerging "smart watch" market. The Apple Watch features Internet connectivity, sensors, and health-tracking apps. But it's safe to say that even smart watches will have their day and eventually make way for ever more integrated sensor technology, not just into clothing, but into the body itself—aka implants.

Regardless of the form of future sensor products, what's really driving the self-tracking revolution is *how the data is used*. What made Fitbit—and similar self-tracking products like the Nike+ wristband and Jawbone UP—different from previous pedometers was the ability to upload your steps and other data to the Internet, and do analysis of it on the Web. In "the cloud," the data can be visualized through graphs and you are given tools to manipulate it, for example to show which time of day you take the most steps. Just as importantly, you can also connect with other people. Donna Allen joined a number of groups on Fitbit, which enabled her to connect to—and be motivated by—similarly health-conscious Fitbit users.

However the future of pedometers and other activity trackers unfolds, Fitbit will adapt. Eric Friedman currently defines Fitbit as a "connecting devices company in the wellness space." But I get the feeling that Eric Friedman would be happiest if the hardware side of his business disappeared altogether, so that Fitbit can simply stick the sensors into your clothes or body. Whatever the case, Friedman assured me that his company will expand into areas of self-tracking "where we can make it more seamless and more ambient."

CHAPTER THREE
DIET WARS: TRACKING FOOD WITH MYFITNESSPAL

There isn't some kind of rigid plan that we ask people to do. It's not like you can never have a piece of chocolate cake again. It's about making your own decisions about what you eat and understanding that there are big ramifications.

Mike Lee, founder of MyFitnessPal

It was the summer of 2003 and Mike Lee, a 32-year-old Silicon Valley marketing executive, was looking forward to his wedding day later that year. The only trouble was, he had put on weight over the summer and didn't want to walk down the aisle with a pudgy tummy. His fiancée also wanted to lose some weight before the big day, so the couple went to see a personal fitness trainer at their local gym, 24-Hour Fitness. At the end of the first session, after Mike Lee and his fiancée had sweated off maybe half a pound, the trainer handed them a small book. It contained calorie counts for about 3,000 foods. "You need to start counting your calories," the trainer advised, tapping the book. "Write down everything that you eat in a notebook."

Mike Lee is a veteran of Silicon Valley. In the early 2000s, he'd worked for Handspring, a manufacturer of PDAs (Personal Digital Assistants) that went on to merge with Palm in 2003.

PDAs were the precursor of the modern smartphone—some of you will remember the Palm Pilot from the early 2000s—and so Lee had gotten an early entry into the world of mobile communications. His first reaction to being told to count calories on paper? There's got to be a digital method! So he immediately threw the calorie counting book away and looked for an online solution. Lee looked at over a dozen existing online calorie counters in the summer of 2003. There was no shortage of online solutions. "But to my amazement," Lee recalled nearly a decade later, "none of them worked the way I thought they should work."

The first thing Mike Lee wanted to change about 2003-era calorie counters was the user experience, which he found frustrating. Many foods were either not available in these products, and so had to be manually input, or if they were available then they were hard to find. "When I was trying to use other products back then," Lee told me over the phone in mid-2013, "the user interfaces were just really cringe-y." He concluded that it was actually easier to write down calorie counts on paper than to use these online products. The second thing he noticed was the lack of intelligence in the online calorie counters of 2003. A simple yet powerful notion, which would become a key feature of MyFitnessPal, was to remember the foods you eat the most. "People tend to eat the same things fairly often," Lee told me, adding that his own breakfast "doesn't vary that much." So he reasoned that an online calorie counter "should just remember what you eat most often and make that easy for you."

Mike Lee left Palm in October 2004 and it was at that point that he began development work on MyFitnessPal. "I started building the diet tracker I really wanted, because I finally had the time to sit down and build it," he told me. It was also a good chance to brush up on his programming skills, being a long-time computing enthusiast and amateur programmer. "I had done a ton of programming when I was young," he said. "I'd started at ten and programmed all the way through high school and college. But it had been a long time ago."

So it was that MyFitnessPal was born, as a side project in 2004 for a slightly overweight Silicon Valley executive. It was officially launched less than a year later, in September 2005. From there it grew into something far beyond a hobby for Mike Lee. By the summer of 2013, MyFitnessPal had attracted over 40 million users and had become the leading calorie counter on the market. But to truly appreciate the scale of what Mike Lee built, we first have to go back to the 1970s—when food tracking was undergoing a revolution.

Diet wars, part I

Calorie counting has had many ups and downs over the years. It's been the subject of furious debates: is it useful at all; how should it be done; are fats more important to track; are carbohydrates the key metric?

Let's start with the basics. What exactly is a calorie and what does it measure? A calorie is a unit of energy. Many of the hundreds of different diets through the years have boiled down to this basic formula: the amount of energy you consume from food must be less than the amount of energy you expend through activity. In other words, the number of calories you eat in a day must be lower than the calories you use up with activity in order for you to lose weight. It was a simple formula and it led to the calorie becoming the default measure of food tracking.

But from the early 1970s, the science of food tracking became more complicated. Dieting became a craze in the 1970s and, in a frantic bid to differentiate themselves, self-proclaimed diet doctors came up with a dizzying number of new theories about how the body processes food. These theories revolved around the three basic components of food: fat, protein, and carbohydrates. Fat and carbohydrates in particular would divide the medical establishment and lead to years of controversy in food tracking.

At first the calorie was still the ultimate food-tracking metric. But the key question became: was it better to minimize calories through controlling fat intake, or carbohydrates? There was a seemingly simple answer to that too. Of the three basic components of food, fat has by far the most calories per gram. According to the American Heart Association (AHA), every one gram of fat is equivalent to nine calories. That makes it over twice as calorie-heavy as carbohydrates and protein, both of which have four calories per gram. The AHA makes it very clear on its website which of the three food components it believes is worst for you:

> *Because fats are so energy-dense, consuming high levels of fat—regardless of the type—can lead to taking in too many calories. That can lead to weight gain or being overweight. Consuming high levels of saturated or trans fats can also lead to heart disease and stroke.*

So not only does a high-fat diet lead to weight problems, according to the AHA, it can lead to heart disease too. That double whammy logic became the foundation of conventional diet programs in the 1970s and 1980s. The key to controlling your calorie intake was to restrict the amount of fat you consumed—that became the accepted wisdom. This approach came to be known as the low-fat diet.

But not everyone subscribed to the low-fat theory. In 1972 Dr. Robert Atkins published his first book, *Dr. Atkins' Diet Revolution*. It followed on from an article in American *Vogue* magazine in 1970, which caused a sensation in the dieting world. Bucking the conventional thinking of the day, Dr. Atkins was recommending a low-carbohydrate approach to dieting. His basic reasoning was that many of the most common foods in the Western diet— breads, grains, starchy vegetables like potatoes—are very high in carbohydrates and therefore high in calories. He also argued that eating a diet high in carbohydrates stimulated appetite. In other words, the more carbs you eat, the hungrier you get, and the more calories you consume in a day.

What Dr. Atkins was advocating was a low-carb diet, which meant that you necessarily had to increase the amount of fats and protein in your diet (if you didn't, you simply wouldn't get enough energy). But this approach had a PR problem: the conventional wisdom that a diet high in fats was high in calories. To get around this, Dr. Atkins made a rule for his new diet: "don't count calories." Instead, he advised dieters to focus on eating "allowed" foods—low-carb foods like steak, eggs, and non-starchy vegetables. High-carbohydrate foods like potatoes, pasta, and breads were forbidden. For followers of the Atkins diet, calorie tracking was put on the back burner.

Dr. Atkins' diet became popular, simply because it worked: people rapidly lost weight on it. But at what long-term cost? Dr. Atkins was a combative personality, and he had developed an intense dislike for the medical establishment since becoming a doctor in the 1950s. His high-fat diet immediately attracted critics in the 1970s. The primary argument against Dr. Atkins was that his diet might help you lose weight in the short term, but it was bad for you in the long run. The high level of fat and protein would lead to heart disease and might also aggravate kidney problems, many physicians maintained.

The dietary views of Dr. Atkins and Dr. Pritikin were diametrically opposed. Dr. Atkins was pushing a high-fat, low-carb, meat-heavy approach; Dr. Pritikin advocated a low-fat, high-carb, plant-based diet.

One of Atkins' most vociferous critics was Dr. Nathan Pritikin, who had actually suffered from heart disease. In 1956, at the age of 41, Dr. Pritikin was diagnosed with coronary artery disease. His total cholesterol reading was over 300 mg/dL, a dangerously high level. He then started a low-fat diet that was high in carbohydrates, and he began running regularly. By January 1960 his total cholesterol was down to 120 mg/dL and he no longer had signs of heart disease. Based on this experience, Dr. Pritikin co-authored a best-selling diet book entitled *The Pritikin Program for Diet and Exercise*. First published in 1979, the book outlined a diet that was "low in fats, cholesterol, protein and highly refined carbohydrates, such as sugars." Conversely, the diet was "high in starches, as part of complex, mostly unrefined carbohydrates." In practical terms, that meant the Pritikin diet was made up of vegetables, potatoes, pastas, breads, and fruit. Small portions of meat were allowed, but not encouraged. Pritikin himself was a vegetarian.

The dietary views of Dr. Atkins and Dr. Pritikin were diametrically opposed. Dr. Atkins was pushing a high-fat, low-carb, meat-heavy approach; Dr. Pritikin advocated a low-fat, high-carb, plant-based diet. Despite the huge gulf in food types recommended by each diet, the Atkins and Pritikin diets did have one thing in common: neither encouraged calorie counting!

Followers of the Pritikin diet were told that there were no restrictions on food quantity: "You can eat as much as you like of many of the permissible foods. All day long, if you wish." Meanwhile, Atkins dieters were told they could have "unrestricted" amounts of meat, fish and shellfish, fowl and eggs (with just a few warnings on certain foods in those wide food groups, such as oysters—which did contain "some carbohydrates"). So during the 1970s and right through to the mid-90s, calorie counting simply wasn't fashionable. In both the popular low-fat diet and the more controversial low-carb approach, calorie counting was discouraged. It was all about *which* food types you could eat—and generally speaking you didn't need to track how much of those foods you ate.

That's not to say that calories weren't still important. Both Atkins and Pritikin believed that weight loss still essentially boiled down to reducing your daily caloric intake. But the two diet doctors had to differentiate their respective diets, from each other and from an increasingly competitive diet marketplace. They also needed a promotional angle that would appeal to a mass audience. The solution for both men was very similar in style, if not the particulars. They simply told their respective followers to eat as much as they liked of the "allowed" foods. Pritikin told people to eat as many carbs as they liked, while Atkins gave the same message about fats. In an era of increasing consumption and sexual promiscuity—the 70s and the early 80s—the two diet doctors cleverly chose to appeal to the appetites of consumers. Eat as much as you like, they cried.

Dr. Atkins even went so far as to crow that his program was much more appetizing. "The advantage of my diet is that it is fun," he told *People* magazine in 1979. "My patients can eat meat or any other main course in whatever quantity they wish, and they never go hungry."

With this background in food tracking, you may be wondering if MyFitnessPal founder Mike Lee had the right motivation in developing a calorie counter in 2004. After all, haven't we just seen that calorie counting isn't necessarily the way to a dieter's heart? But the question is moot, because what Lee ended up building tracked more than just calories. It also enabled people to track intake of fats, carbohydrates, protein, salt levels, sugar, and much more. Mike Lee left it up to his users to choose what they tracked. He just gave them the right tool.

MyFitnessPal goes mobile

In August 2009, after five years of part-time work building up MyFitnessPal, Mike Lee finally decided to take the big step and quit his day job. His brother Al Lee also joined him as a full-time employee of MyFitnessPal. It was to be a turning point for the young company. It was also a key period for the consumer health technology market. As we saw in the previous chapter, it was the year that the Fitbit activity tracker began shipping. Other health-focused websites and apps began to appear too. The primary reason for the increased popularity of health apps like Fitbit and MyFitnessPal in 2009 was the smartphone.

The second half of 2008 saw two milestones on the Internet landscape, which ultimately propelled the smartphone into the limelight. Following on from the launch of the first-generation iPhone in 2007, in July 2008 Apple launched the second-generation (dubbed the iPhone 3G) and—just as importantly—an App Store. The first Android-powered smartphone to be released came just a few months later, in October 2008. So coming into the New Year, 2009, the market was primed for a new way to use the Internet: smartphone apps. In an August 2009 blog post announcing that he and Al were devoting themselves to

MyFitnessPal full-time, Mike Lee noted that they were already working on "an iPhone app which we modestly think will be the best calorie counting app in the app store." The iPhone app was duly launched in December 2009 and it led to a surge in popularity for MyFitnessPal. Like many health-related Internet products, MyFitnessPal was a perfect match for the smartphone. "You want to be tracking when you're actually eating," explained Mike Lee in our 2013 interview, "and that's when you're out and about. So, mobile was critical to us."

I was a relative latecomer to MyFitnessPal. I started to use it in early 2013, when I began a new diet—a low-carb one, as it happens. I used the MyFitnessPal iPhone app to enter my food for a period of about three months. I focused mainly on counting carbohydrate intake each day, since that was what my new diet required. But I found myself interested in all of the different food data, for comparative reasons. For example, I could compare the calories that MyFitnessPal said I consumed with the calories that Fitbit said I expended. Every time I ate something, it took a couple of minutes at most to enter the data into MyFitnessPal.

I don't think I would have used the product at all if it wasn't for the mobile app. It would have been too much of a hassle for me to open my computer and enter the data multiple times a day. But I carry my smartphone around with me everywhere, so it was easy to track my food intake. That, in a nutshell, is why MyFitnessPal became so popular in 2010 and beyond: it was a killer smartphone app waiting to happen.

It became even easier when MyFitnessPal added barcode scanning to its Android app in November 2010 (the iPhone app got this in July 2011). The feature uses the smartphone's camera to take a photo of a product barcode, which the MyFitnessPal app would attempt to match to a product in its food database. If a match was found, which in my experience was more often than not, the food would be automatically added to your meal. In my discussions with Mike Lee, I was somewhat surprised to learn that the data doesn't come from the food manufacturers. "We don't go direct to the food manufacturers to get the food data, in most cases," said Lee. Rather, it is crowdsourced. In other words, MyFitnessPal's users upload the data and check it for accuracy.

One of the items I scanned into my food log every now and then was Kraft's Philadelphia Regular Cream Cheese Spread. The calorie, carb, fat, and other nutrition data for this product was member-submitted. It had "two confirmations" when I last checked, meaning that two people had reviewed the data against the product's label and deemed it correct. It's easy enough to check yourself, since many countries legally require food manufacturers to have a nutrition facts label on the packaging. The one thing to be wary of is that some nutrition labels can be misleading or wrong. The US Food and Drug Administration (FDA) states on its website: "Manufacturers are responsible for the accuracy of the nutrition labeling values on their products." The FDA does random sampling for accuracy and it will prosecute violations, but it simply doesn't have the resources to check everything.

The barcode scanning feature led to more MyFitnessPal users adding data to an already impressive database of food information. MyFitnessPal's food database has been critical to its success over the years. Mike Lee realized very early on that in a food tracking app, there's nothing more frustrating for a user than not finding an item—because then they'd need to check the food packaging and manually input the data. What should be a quick one-minute update becomes a five or even ten-minute time suck. So top of mind for Mike Lee when he began developing MyFitnessPal in 2004 was building up a large food database.

He began by manually adding the data himself, using product information from food manufacturers and retailers where available. In September 2007, Lee blogged: "Last night, I was able to add nutritional information for the entire Starbucks menu and all Amy's Kitchen products to the food database. My goal is to more than triple the size of the current food database by the end of the year." But he also realized that MyFitnessPal would only truly scale if he called on his users to help, in other words, crowdsource it by enabling MyFitnessPal's users to input and check data. The alternatives were to get the data from open food nutrition databases or directly pipe it from food manufacturers. However, there wasn't a comprehensive open database of barcodes that MyFitnessPal could tap into, and getting the data from food manufacturers was far too much work. Besides, if their own users entered the data then MyFitnessPal would own it.

One of the defining characteristics of so-called "social" software—like Facebook and Twitter—is that the value of the business is almost all derived from the amount and quality of user data in its databases. MyFitnessPal is no exception, so Mike Lee was very smart to go the crowdsourcing route. Everything its users enter into MyFitnessPal's food database belongs to MyFitnessPal.

Still, it was no easy task to build up the food database. If he wasn't adding new foods himself, Mike Lee spent his time checking the accuracy on user submissions. It was a chicken-and-egg situation in 2005 when MyFitnessPal launched because there needed to be enough food data to grow its user base, but there was a danger that early users would be frustrated by lack of data and immediately quit.

Lee got around this dilemma with some ingenious solutions, such as letting MyFitnessPal's earliest users check data accuracy with just one click of a button. This was the birth of the "confirmations" mentioned earlier, in the Kraft cream cheese example. If a user came across a food that had member-supplied data, next to it was a message (Is this data accurate?) along with two buttons (yes and no).

Fortunately for Mike Lee, enough of the early users glanced down to their food packaging to check the MyFitnessPal data. So gradually, from 2005 onward, the MyFitnessPal database began to fill out. MyFitnessPal has come a long way since 2005. Nowadays, with tens of millions of users, it has built-in quality control. "We have a million QA people now," Lee said, chuckling … probably with relief that he no longer needs to check the data himself.

Diet wars, part II

When we left our two diet doctors, Dr. Atkins and Dr. Pritikin, they were both espousing an "all you can eat" approach to their followers. There were many diets to choose from during this period, the late 70s and early 80s, including wacky ones such as fruitarian and the cabbage soup diet (the names tell you all you need to know about what you could eat). But the Atkins and Pritikin programs represented the two main approaches to dieting.

Of the two, the low-fat diet epitomized by Pritikin had the huge advantage of adhering to conventional wisdom. As a result, despite the efforts of the voluble Dr. Robert Atkins, the low-fat diet dominated right through the 80s and into the 90s. Standards organizations such as the American Heart Association (AHA) and American Diabetes Association (ADA) strongly advocated the low-fat approach (most of them still do, to this day). As for calorie counting, it was still practiced— but it was widely viewed as more important to monitor the fat content of foods. Fat counts, not calories, was the metric of the day.

In the mid-90s, carbohydrates became the focus again thanks to the Glycemic Index. Created in 1981 by Dr. Thomas Wolever and Dr. David Jenkins at the University of Toronto, the Glycemic Index (usually abbreviated to GI) measures how quickly your blood sugar levels rise after eating carbohydrates. The index uses a scale from 0–100, with 100 equivalent to pure glucose. The lower the score for a particular food, the longer it takes for your body to process it. The theory is that low-glycemic foods better regulate your insulin levels, which in turn enables you to control your appetite. A score of 70 and above is considered high and means that your blood sugar level will rise very quickly after you eat. The staple breakfast cereal of cornflakes, for example, has a shockingly high GI level of 93. That means it's almost the same as eating a bowl of white sugar for breakfast! On the other hand, boiled whole-wheat spaghetti has a GI rating of 42. So it was foods such as this that made up low-glycemic diets, which became popular in the mid-1990s.

The South Beach Diet is one of the better known low-GI diets still in use today.

The low-glycemic theory was similar to that of the low-carb diets of Dr. Atkins and others. The goal in both cases was to regulate your hormones, principally insulin, so that your blood sugar levels were under control and you won't get hungry so often. Where the two dietary approaches differed was that low-glycemic foods are often still high in carbohydrates, which earned such foods the nickname of "good carbs." It was the speed at which carbs were processed in your body, not the number of carbs, which was important for low-GI diets. Dr. Atkins rejected that theory—for him, there was no such thing as good carbs.

So-called "whole grains" became very fashionable in the 1990s and beyond for those on low-GI diets. Many of these foods, for example the whole-wheat spaghetti mentioned above, were high in carbs but low GI. In effect, following a low-glycemic diet meant that you could eat a wider range of foods than on an Atkins-style low-carb diet. In particular, you could eat grains and breads—as long as they were made from the wholesome-sounding "whole grains." As a result of the GI, counting calories began to make a comeback in the mid- to late 1990s. That's because counting carbohydrates and fat was no longer sufficient to get a full picture of your daily food intake. Calorie counting by itself didn't solve the problem either, so a common approach for diet doctors and weight-loss companies in the mid-90s onward was to create a proprietary "formula" that incorporated GI levels. Usually these formulas were founded on calories, which had the effect of making calorie counting trendy again. For example, Weight Watchers launched a points system in 1997 that was GI-friendly, but almost entirely based on calories (I'll explore Weight Watchers in more detail in the next chapter, which is about tracking weight).

However, within a decade the calorie itself would come under pressure as a metric of food consumption. In 2007, science writer Gary Taubes published a book called *Good Calories, Bad Calories*. The book, weighing in at over 500 pages, argued that calorie counting was the wrong approach to understanding weight gain. Instead, wrote Taubes, it all came down to carbohydrate counting. He went further: over-consumption of carbohydrates was the primary cause of the obesity epidemic. He argued that the key to weight gain was insulin, the hormone in our bodies that regulates blood sugar levels. Taubes presented a very detailed analysis of medical research showing that if you eat high-carb foods, the body produces too much insulin, which leads to sugar levels rising rapidly, then falling just as rapidly, which in turn causes the body to crave more food—and so on, in a vicious circle. The upshot is weight gain. The solution? Eat fewer carbs. "The fewer carbohydrates we consume," concluded Taubes, "the leaner we will be."

Taubes' book changed the way the diet industry thought about weight loss. It was the follow-up to a *New York Times* magazine article he'd written in 2002, which caused a sensation. Entitled "What If It's All Been a Big Fat Lie?", the article argued that the low-fat dietary approach endorsed by the American medical establishment over the past twenty years had been completely wrong-headed. Dr. Atkins had been right all along, the article stated. Unfortunately for Dr. Atkins, he didn't live to benefit from this vindication. He died less than a year later, in April 2003—ironically under a cloud of suspicion that he was obese at the time.

Sometimes it's not the carbohydrates or calories that we're concerned with when it comes to monitoring our health. Salt is a popular bad boy in the modern diet, because too much salt in our diet can raise blood pressure. Indeed, different diets emphasize different risks. The Paleo diet has become very trendy in the early part of the 21st century, as a movement against processed foods. It was named after the diet that our Paleolithic ancestors presumably would have eaten, over 10,000 years ago. Paleolithic hunter-gatherers subsisted on meat, vegetables, and some fruit. So the Paleo diet outlaws any type of food that our ancestors would not have consumed. That means everything that the Neolithic agricultural revolution brought us, especially grains and sugars. The basic premise of the Paleo diet is that our bodies have not fully adapted to processed foods like grains and sugars, since for over 99% of the period of our evolution we haven't consumed such foods.

Personally, I find the premise of the Paleo diet rather shaky. Yes, our ancestors 10,000 years ago got by just fine on this diet. But they also had a far lower life expectancy and, as hunter-gatherers, lived an entirely different way from us. Also, nobody really knows how our bodies evolve over time. In terms of its foods, the Paleo diet is similar to an Atkins-style diet in that much of it is low in carbohydrates. However, the Paleo diet is a lot more restrictive. For example, unlike most low-carb diets, the Paleo diet has deemed that legumes are bad. Legumes are foods that come from a pod and include beans, peas, lentils, soybeans and peanuts. So why are they bad? According to Loren Cordain, author of *The Paleo Diet*, "Most legumes in their mature state are non-digestible and/or toxic to most mammals when eaten in even moderate quantities." Legumes are "non-digestible and/ or toxic" because—like grains—they contain phytic acid, which prevents you from absorbing nutrients.

But different diets work for different people. As a type 1 diabetic, I found that a low-carb diet that regulates my blood sugar levels is best for me. However, I didn't just start a low-carb diet and accept it as the best, even though there's no shortage of books and websites telling me it is. Using MyFitnessPal and my blood glucose meter, I tracked the foods I ate over a period of a few months, paying special attention to the effect of carbohydrates on my body. So I didn't just accept the literature, I tested for myself if the low-carb diet was effective for me.

> **By all means try out the latest fashionable diet, but make sure you track the results.**

Perhaps the Paleo diet will work better for you, or maybe one of the low-fat diets still recommended to this day by the American Heart Association. Or vegetarianism. The purpose of my book is not to recommend any particular diet or course of action. It's to emphasize that you should find out—of your own accord—what works best for you. Tracking your food intake is an effective way of doing that. By all means try out the latest fashionable diet, but make sure you track the results.

So what to count when you're tracking your food intake? The short answer is that it depends on your diet. If you're on a low-carb diet, then it obviously makes sense to keep track of your daily carbs. If you still like your wholegrain breads and Italian pasta dishes (and your body can process them well), then counting calories is a good way to go. As long as you realize that there isn't an exact correlation between calories in and calories out. The food tracking tools of today cater for it all. While MyFitnessPal began as a simple calorie counter, it now also enables you to count your daily carbs, fat, protein, cholesterol, sodium, sugars, and fiber.

It all comes back to the power of knowledge. Tracking your food, at least for a short time, tells you what you're putting into your body every day. Some of those measures will be more important to you than others. For me, carbs is what I focus on. I do keep an eye on calories too, but mainly because that allows me to cross-check my calories-in (food) with calories-out (activity) figures, which I can track with a pedometer device like Fitbit or Nike FuelBand.

Different strokes for different folks

When MyFitnessPal released its iPhone app in December 2009, it enabled people to track their food on the go. I asked founder Mike Lee what he's learned since then about how to track food intake. The first thing a new MyFitnessPal user should do, replied Lee, is "track everything." But it's OK to estimate food data, he added: "It doesn't have to be perfect. The most important thing is just keep tracking." He also advises not to worry about missing the odd meal. "The more you do it," he said about food tracking, "the easier it becomes and the more of a habit it becomes. Basically, the longer you stick with it, the more success you're going to have." Another tip Mike Lee offered is to enter your food before you eat, not after. That's where the smartphone app really helps, because it takes a couple of minutes at most to enter this data. The benefit of doing it before you eat is that you can make adjustments if a food you're about to consume is high in calories, or carbohydrates, or whatever your key metric is.

Some of the power users of MyFitnessPal use the app to plan their meals throughout the day, although many people will prefer less structure. Mike Lee himself prefers a more flexible approach. "There isn't some kind of rigid plan that we ask people to do," he told me. "It's not like you can never have a piece of chocolate cake again. It's about making your own decisions about what you eat and understanding that there are big ramifications." In his own life, as a startup CEO, he often needs to go to industry events. Such events tend to serve nibbles along with alcohol and so are likely to push his calorie count up for that day. "So I'll go lighter on lunch," explained Lee, "or I'll go for a run in the afternoon to try to burn off some extra calories." So for Mike Lee, his app gives him an understanding of what tradeoffs he can make every day about his food and exercise mix. "It's just really empowering," he said. "You feel like you're in control of what you want and goals that you're trying to achieve and that's kind of what I like about it."

Ultimately the benefit of food tracking apps like MyFitnessPal is that they help you make better food choices, whatever flavor of diet you subscribe to. "Everybody can benefit from eating better," Mike Lee remarked. "Until recently, we didn't have the tools to make the [food] information we need easily accessible." For example, Lee—who still uses calories as his primary measure—stopped using mayonnaise on his sandwiches after discovering how many calories it had. "One tablespoon of mayonnaise has 90 calories. Before I started calorie counting, I had no idea that was the case. Whereas mustard has five calories. So I just stopped using mayonnaise." This is the kind of food knowledge, says Mike Lee, that stays with you and helps you make better daily decisions.

It's important to note that it's not scientific knowledge that Mike Lee is referring to, but self-knowledge. The diet industry is one of the most confusing and contradictory around. When two diametrically opposed diets—low fat and low carb—both have science "facts" to back them up, it's no surprise that most people have little clue which foods are truly healthy. In the final analysis, food facts may not matter that much. Mike Lee to this day emphasizes calorie counting in his own ongoing weight maintenance plan, even though counting carbs is more in fashion now. Whichever metric you use, monitoring your food intake will at the very least make you more mindful of what you're eating and the impact it has on your weight.

I myself agree with Dr. Atkins and Gary Taubes that it's carbohydrates that ultimately lead to weight gain. That said, I don't do a low-carb diet because of weight issues. I do it because I'm a type 1 diabetic, and reducing carbohydrates is the most effective way for me to control my daily blood sugar levels. I have lost a bit of weight too, but if anything I'd prefer to put some of it back on. If I wasn't a type 1 diabetic, then I probably wouldn't be on a low-carb diet. I don't have a tendency to put on a lot of weight, so I'd be able to get by on a regular carb-loaded diet if it wasn't for my diabetes.

Atkins was a fairly big man, around 6 feet and 200 pounds. Taubes too is a big man, at 6 feet 3 inches and over 200 pounds. Atkins did the low-carb diet because it was his most effective way of losing weight and keeping it off. Taubes had a similar experience. But Nathan Pritikin—described in his biography as "a thin, wiry man, no more than five feet, eight inches tall"—did the complete opposite diet and he too managed to stay slim. Different strokes for different folks is a cliché that is apt here. It needn't even be about one's height or body shape. Perhaps it's the way your body processes food.

A journalist friend of Gary Taubes, John Horgan from *Scientific American* magazine, follows a carb-heavy diet but has a lower BMI than Taubes: "I'm 1.85 meters [6 feet, 1 inch] tall. I eat lots of carbs, including pasta, bread, rice, potatoes, cookies, cake, pie, and three teaspoons of sugar in coffee at least twice a day. I weigh 77 kilograms [170 pounds]. I'm just one of those lucky folks whose genes let them chow down carbs without getting fat."

There is no one diet to fit all. Each of us is different. What's more, our circumstances change over time—from experience, I can tell you that getting type 1 diabetes will make you change your diet! Ultimately, the only way you'll find out which type of diet is effective for you is by testing them and tracking your progress. Whether you use a smartphone calorie (or carb, or salt, etc.) counter like MyFitnessPal, or whether you use good old paper and pen, it doesn't matter, although the technology in MyFitnessPal does make things easier. The main point though is to test for yourself what works.

But how often do you need to use a tool like MyFitnessPal? From my own usage, I can attest that although it only takes five to ten minutes a day in total, it does take a conscious effort to do every update. Also, some updates are difficult to make, for example, when you're eating out and you don't know exactly what's in the foods you're consuming.

Many people use MyFitnessPal intensely for a short period, then stop. I was one of those users. I began my low-carb diet in mid-March 2013 and started using MyFitnessPal at the same time. It helped me immensely in knowing how many carbs I was consuming every day, as well as avoiding eating foods that were high carb. After a few months of using MyFitnessPal regularly, I came to an understanding of what my average daily carb consumption was. At that point I stopped using the app. That's because what I eat every day is fairly consistent: I have a salmon omelette most mornings for breakfast, a salad for lunch, a meat and green veggies dinner. Even when I deviate from my eating routines, I know which foods to avoid now, and so I don't feel I need to enter the data into MyFitnessPal.

Mike Lee admitted that this kind of usage is fairly common for his app. Some users, he said, "use the app for a while, maybe they'll hit their goal weight, for example, and they'll feel like they don't need to track anymore. But then, oftentimes they'll come back a few months later for a little clean-up." MyFitnessPal sees a broad pattern of behavior, said Lee. "Some people calling it off, some people doing it every single day. It really depends on what the user is looking for." Even Mike Lee himself doesn't use MyFitnessPal for every single meal. "I log most of the time," he told me. "There are some meals that I'll skip. But in those cases, I still use the general knowledge that I've gained from the app."

On that last point, I must correct Mike Lee. It's not "general" knowledge he's gained from tracking his foods on the app he created—it's the knowledge of what is best for his own body.

CHAPTER FOUR
THE TAO OF WEIGHT TRACKING

The tracking, the paying attention, just seems to me like it enforces more mindfulness and more compassion for myself.

Amelia Greenhall, weight tracker

Just as there are many different ways to track your food input, there are many different theories about how to lose weight. But at least weight tracking itself is simple. All you need to do is hop on a scale and see how many pounds you weigh (or kilograms, for those of us in the former British Empire). What's more, just as Fitbit did with the pedometer, the modern scale is an Internet-connected device. Fitbit itself began selling a scale in 2012, called the Aria. It got the idea from a French company called Withings, which released the world's first Internet scale in 2009.

Amelia Greenhall began tracking her weight in January 2007 when she was a junior studying electrical engineering at Vanderbilt University, Nashville. She wasn't even overweight. But with the tall and sturdy frame of a female basketball player, Greenhall felt self-conscious about her body. She somehow felt too heavy—not "light and fit" enough, as she put it. So, inspired by a book entitled *The Hacker's Diet*, Greenhall set out to lose a few pounds.

At first, her method of tracking her weight loss was low-tech. "Every day I woke up and stepped on the scale naked, right after I peed," she recalled. "It was just a $20 digital scale with half-pound precision, but it was accurate enough. Then I wrote it down in a buff Moleskine notebook that sat on my dresser, bookmarked with the pencil." Almost every day for the next two years, Greenhall recorded her weight in the notebook. Every few weeks she would transfer the figures into a spreadsheet and, prompted by *The Hacker's Diet*, plot the ten-day running average. Greenhall kept up this manual method of weight tracking until late 2011, when she bought an Internet-connected Withings scale.

Looking at Amelia Greenhall now, via a video Skype call in late April 2013, she is the picture of smiling health. The 26-year-old's face is tanned and her long black hair is tied in a sporty ponytail. She looks fit and happy. I know from reading her blog that she's vegetarian and leads an active outdoors lifestyle with her husband, Adam. Yet despite this healthy life and seemingly having little reason to worry about her weight, she continues to track it. That's because this form of self-tracking has become a prime motivator for her.

At first, weight tracking for Amelia Greenhall was about losing a few pounds. But it soon became more than that. It turned into an ongoing experiment in self-reflection. Once she had shed the extra pounds, Greenhall realized that she wanted to continue because weight tracking was helping her understand her body. "I wanted to get in touch with my body," she explained, adding that weight tracking felt similar to practicing yoga—which she also did in college. Weight tracking was now about increasing her self-awareness and finding ways to feel happy in her skin.

> "I was trying to do the least amount of tracking that would give me actionable knowledge."

Even though weight was Greenhall's primary body measurement, she tracked other things too. In particular she monitored how often she did certain activities, such as going for a bike ride or a run. She was looking for correlations between her activities and her weight. She hastened to point out that she never obsessed over details. "I was trying to do the least amount of tracking that would give me actionable knowledge," she told me. Her modus operandi was to experiment with tracking various activities—even things like going to parties—to see what affected her weight. One of her goals was to find activities she enjoyed doing, but which also helped her control her weight. Ultimately, she wanted to make changes to her lifestyle and find fun activities that she could maintain for the rest of her life. "I knew that I really liked climbing," she reflected in 2013, "and I really, really liked bike commuting." So she tracked those activities to see how they impacted her weight.

Over the years, Greenhall has found that her weight is a great barometer for her overall health and enjoyment of life. "If it goes too high or drops too low, I know that it's a trigger to inspect my life and make sure I'm eating, sleeping, and exercising well." But if the ten-day running average stays within a couple of pounds of her goal, then she's happy. In this sense, tracking weight has become an early warning system for Greenhall. "It'll show problems in me not taking care of myself sooner than I would've noticed or admitted to myself," she noted.

Surprisingly, Greenhall isn't that concerned about how regularly she weighs herself. In fact there are large gaps in her weight tracking since 2007, in particular during the times she's traveled. But it's the trend line that matters to Greenhall and she has been able to paper in the travel gaps. In 2009, she went camping for four months with her husband, Adam. She didn't weigh herself during that time, but later she was easily able to pick up the trend line again.

For Greenhall, numbers aren't as important as how she feels. Her weight readings, in particular the moving average, give her something to measure. But they must always be cross-checked with her feelings. When Greenhall started weight tracking in 2007, she set a target weight. But she soon learned to take the approach of "I'm going to go in this direction and explore, see what feels good" rather than "I'm going to hit this weight no matter what." What she calls her "natural weight" turned out to be lower than she initially thought. "I thought maybe I would go from 180 to 150, which is where I had been in high school." But she eventually settled at around 140 pounds.

She was also surprised to discover that a certain amount of weight gain was a good thing. During the summer of 2012 she did a lot of mountain climbing and gained muscle mass. But once she figured out why her weight had gone up—and that it was a good thing, because it was muscle and not fat—she relaxed. "The tracking, the paying attention, just seems to me like it enforces more mindfulness and more compassion for myself ... and how I'm feeling."

Greenhall is obviously taking care of herself, because nowadays her primary goal with weight tracking is maintenance. "In 2007 I used weight tracking to make changes in my lifestyle in order to lose weight," she said. "But for the past few years my goal has been to stay the same." In other words, she self-tracks to stay healthy and happy.

Social support with Weight Watchers

Of course not everyone is as happy about their weight as Amelia Greenhall. In the Western world there is almost an epidemic of overweight people. According to World Health Organization (WHO) figures at time of writing, a staggering 67% of Americans are classified as overweight. Worse, 34% of all Americans are obese—which basically means very overweight.

WHO defines an overweight person as someone with a body mass index (BMI) of 25 or over. An obese person is someone who has a BMI of 30 or over. BMI is simply an estimate of your body fat—between 18.5 and 24.9 is considered "normal." The BMI formula has just two variables: your weight and your height. The formula is kg/m²: weight in kilograms divided by the square of the height. Generally speaking, the higher your BMI, the higher your risk of some of the body systems diseases we've discussed in this book already: type 2 diabetes, heart disease, certain cancers.

The BMI index isn't perfect, because weight doesn't always correlate with height. For example athletes and people with a muscular build often have a high BMI, because a good portion of their weight is made up of muscle. So just because they have a higher BMI than average doesn't necessarily mean they are overweight or obese. BMI also doesn't fully factor in that men and women have different makeups in terms of body fat.

For these reasons, a new measure called "body fat percentage" is often viewed as a better indicator of healthy weight than BMI. Modern Internet-connected scales, such as the Withings and the Fitbit Aria, tend to emphasize body fat percentage over BMI. Partly that's because they've come up with clever new software to measure it. Both Withings and Fitbit pass a tiny electrical current through your bare feet when you step on the scales. Jonathan Choquel from Withings explained: "As electricity doesn't behave the same when it goes through fat, muscle, bone or fluids, our engineers were able to build an algorithm that extrapolates your body's opposition to the current and provides you with a fat-lean ratio." It's a nifty bit of technology, although in my experience these measurements can vary significantly from day to day.

Overweight formulas for BMI are the same for both men and women, but with body fat percentage it's different. Men are considered to be overweight if their body fat is 21–25% of their entire weight. They're labeled obese if they are over 25%. For women the threshold is higher, with 31–33% body fat to weight ratio considered overweight, and over 33% obese. In other words, women naturally have a higher density of body fat than men. Once again, though, athletes and other very fit people don't easily fit into these formulas. Fitbit even has two settings for its scale: "regular" (the default, for normal people) and "lean" (for professional athletes). The algorithm for "lean" people adjusts their body fat percentage down, to account for the extra muscle.

Because it's simpler and the formula is the same for both sexes, the BMI is the measure most often cited in medical reports about obesity. Using the BMI, the World Health Organization rates the US as having the sixth highest overweight figures in the world. Only five much smaller countries have more than 67% of their population classed as overweight: American Samoa,

Kiribati, French Polynesia, Saudi Arabia, and Panama. However, some larger European countries don't fare much better: Germany is at 66.5%, and the UK and Northern Ireland at 61%. By comparison, Asian countries are much skinnier. Only 19% of China's population is overweight and 13.5% of Indonesia's. India has the lowest percentage of overweight citizens in the world, at 4.5%.

The news doesn't get any better for the US in obesity figures, defined as a BMI of 30 or above. According to the WHO, 34% of Americans are defined as obese—over a third of the population! That places the US ninth on the global list, behind a string of tiny Pacific islands plus Saudi Arabia and Panama. Germany, incidentally, has much less of a problem with obesity than the US, with only 13% of its population classified as "obese." The percentage of obese citizens in the UK and Northern Ireland is nearly 23%.

The US figures from the WHO relate to 2006, the most recent figures available at time of writing. The National Health and Nutrition Examination Survey of 2009–2010 has fairly similar findings, though, with 35.7% of US men and women aged twenty and over classified as obese. Even more worryingly, that same survey found that nearly 17% of US children and adolescents were obese.

With these statistics in mind, it's no surprise that losing weight is the most popular health issue in the US. Yet it's also one of the hardest things for many people to do: to lose weight, and keep it off. There's a difference between the sexes, for a start. Men tend to have a higher metabolism than women and therefore burn calories faster. Weight loss also has a number of societal factors. How easy it is for you to lose weight depends on your age, economic status, where you live and a whole host of other variables. There's even been talk in the media of a "fat gene" that predisposes you to gain weight, although it is unproven at this time.

Tracking weight is relatively easy for Amelia Greenhall, simply because she's a young, active, relatively well-off urban dweller. But for many people, tracking weight is an exercise in frustration and failure. In a nutshell, they need support. Encouragement from others, particularly people who are also tracking the same thing, always helps. But it's particularly the case with weight, because of the difficulties in losing or maintaining weight. That's where organizations like Weight Watchers come in.

Weight Watchers was the first weight loss program to go beyond diet advice and offer an almost religious sense of community as well. It's not just a diet, goes the PR, it's "a healthy way to live." Tracking is a core part of the Weight Watchers experience, because you are actively measuring and monitoring your weight. Not only that, you also regularly report your weight to fellow members of Weight Watchers, which is ultimately what makes Weight Watchers work: social support.

Weight Watchers began in 1961 as a support group for overweight women. It was started by Jean Nidetch, a 5-foot, 7-inch, 38-year-old Brooklyn woman who at the time weighed 214 pounds (that's a BMI of 32.5, so the WHO would have classified her as obese). The group met every week for check-ins, reaching 40 participants within a couple of months. Nidetch herself successfully lost 72 pounds by October 1962. She went on to incorporate Weight Watchers in 1963.

Nidetch realized that the way to lose weight was twofold. First, an easy way to track your progress. For this, Weight Watchers eventually developed a points system. In the beginning, though, it was simply a set of diets that you either adhered to or not. But tracking alone wasn't sufficient because too often people fall off the wagon, as Nidetch herself had done in the past. So the second key to Weight Watchers was its social support system—getting help and encouragement from other people in the same boat. Using the power of social networking in a pre-Internet age, Weight Watchers became very effective at helping its members change their eating and activity habits.

When Nidetch started Weight Watchers, she and her fellow members had a limited knowledge of why people put on weight. In Nidetch's case, she confessed she was overweight because she binged on certain foods—in particular, cookies. Many of the early members of Weight Watchers had the same problem, binge eating, so in effect the organization began as a kind of Alcoholics Anonymous. Its members had simply substituted over-eating for drinking too much.

Weight Watchers now runs 50,000 face-to-face meetings every week, across the world. The goal of the meetings is to provide support to members, with the idea that it will lead to lasting change. Meetings are typically held in community centers, schools, offices, malls, and churches. Each meeting has a leader, usually a Weight Watchers success story. The leaders are notoriously underpaid, which has led to varying quality. But regardless, these meetings historically have worked for Weight Watchers. It all comes down to one thing: peer pressure. We normally associate peer pressure with bad things, such as bullying or groupthink. But Weight Watchers has shown that peer pressure can be a very positive thing if it provides regular motivation to change and a sense of community. One member said about the meetings that they give her "a weekly reboot to stay focused and motivated."

But while the meetings generally have a supportive atmosphere, there is a dangerous underlying assumption: if you aren't succeeding in losing weight, then you're not using the program correctly—or worse, you're cheating. This philosophy was borne out in an advert I saw recently on the Weight Watchers AUNZ Facebook page, which stated: "If you sort of track, you will sort of lose weight." Some people respond well to that kind of social pressure to do everything by the book, including tracking everything you eat accurately. Some people can't cope with the peer pressure, or more commonly find that something in the Weight Watchers program doesn't work for their particular circumstances.

What about online communities, such as MyFitnessPal's message boards: can they provide a free alternative to Weight Watchers? There's no doubt online communities do provide support, but they also have much less structure than a commercial program like Weight Watchers. In short, it's easier to cheat yourself if you rely on self-help communities. You're likely to come across dozens of theories in an online forum, because online communities tend to be both more vocal and more extreme in opinions.

The core message of this book is that everyone is unique; therefore, tracking must be tailored to your own body. But you may also need support, especially with a goal as tough as losing weight. While there is a danger of groupthink when doing a program like Weight Watchers—in other words, there is a central dogma and it is enforced by the majority—the benefits often outweigh that danger. The fact is that the social support Weight Watchers provides has been proven to work for many people over the years.

Is it better to sign up with Weight Watchers, an established and successful social support system, or go it alone like Amelia Greenhall? Weight Watchers has funded a number of research studies that (surprise, surprise) conclude that it is better to do its program. The biggest was a study published in *JAMA: The Journal of the American Medical Association* in 2003. In a two-year randomized clinical trial, 309 participants were assigned to either a self-help program or to a commercial weight loss program (specifically, Weight Watchers). The self-help program consisted of two twenty-minute counseling sessions with a nutritionist, along with self-help resources. The Weight Watchers program featured a food plan, an activity plan, and weekly support meetings. The results of the study, after two years, showed "the structured commercial weight loss program provided modest weight loss, but more than self-help." The key word there is "modest." The Weight Watchers group had lost an average of 11 pounds after one year and 6.6 pounds after two years. The self-help group had lost an average of 3 pounds after a year, but had pretty much returned to their start weight by the end of two years.

I don't find those conclusions convincing. There isn't enough of a difference to suggest that choosing Weight Watchers is the way to go. So what are the practical pros and cons? The clear advantage of Weight Watchers is that you are motivated by your peer group. If you go the independent route, you don't necessarily get that support—although, in Amelia's case, her husband shares her fondness for outdoor pursuits. However, going it alone means that you get to tailor a program that suits your individual needs. It's also going to be a lot cheaper and may lead to fun lifestyle changes.

Amelia's method

For Amelia Greenhall, biking became a key way for her to lose weight, and have fun at the same time. But if it wasn't for self-tracking, she wouldn't have kept up the biking. She first discovered the joys of biking one summer in Germany while on an internship during her college years. There, she would bike to and from work and take weekend bike tours. This experience motivated her to become a bike commuter back in the US. But initially she found it difficult. "It was hard to get started," she reflected. "It's not an easy thing to do to get out there in traffic and to learn all the right tools and skills." However, she found that tracking her biking activity helped her to persist. "Tracking it and seeing the quantitative difference in how I was feeling and my weight, that really encouraged me to keep doing it, stick with it through the hard part. Now, there's no way I would give it up because it's so fun. It's such a great way of living for me."

I asked Amelia what she'd recommend to people who want to try losing weight on their own. Not everyone can afford Weight Watchers and the peer pressure puts other people off. So how can one lose weight, using self-tracking?

According to Amelia Greenhall, all you need to start tracking your weight is a set of scales and a paper notebook. After you've been tracking for a week or two, calculate a ten-day running average of your weight. This can be done using a spreadsheet and a template that you can easily find with a Google search. "I've done this a few times with coaching various people," said Greenhall. She even got her father to adopt her self-tracking method. After watching her dad take up biking, she encouraged him to start a Google Docs spreadsheet in order to track his weight and the ten-day running average. He also tracked how many miles he biked each day and made notes if, for example, he'd gone to a barbecue and eaten more than usual. According to Greenhall, this kind of self-reflection is essential to getting started on tracking your weight. "Start logging anything you feel is significant about what you ate, how you exercised, how you felt and your weight." She paused. "Then calculate the ten-day running average, either daily or every week or so."

The important thing, she emphasized, is to approach your weight tracking as an experiment. "What if I do this? What happens? Try not to take it very seriously, just focus on the overall trend." The day-to-day numbers don't matter, Greenhall insisted. It's better to look at the trend line. Why ten days for the average? Greenhall replied that it needs to be longer than a week to smooth out variations, such as a changed routine in the weekend. It's the variations that tend to cause stress when trying to lose weight. "You're trying to remove variation and get information back about yourself that can help you make decisions," said Greenhall. On the other hand, longer than two weeks doesn't give you information quickly enough if you make a change in your diet or lifestyle.

> **The important thing is to approach your weight tracking as an experiment.**

Interestingly, Weight Watchers founder Jean Nidetch also advocated not obsessing over the daily weight readings. In her first book, *The Story of Weight Watchers*, she wrote that members should only weigh themselves once a week. Because one's weight fluctuates from day to day, people were setting themselves up for disappointment if they did daily weigh-ins. Weekly weigh-ins, she concluded, are "much easier on the nerves."

Another benefit of tracking the ten-day running average is that it makes tracking your weight a more relaxing affair. If you're aggressively following a diet to lose 10 or 20 pounds over a short amount of time, then the day-to-day numbers will be more relevant. But if you're taking a less intense approach, or simply want to maintain your weight long-term, then the ten-day running average is all you need.

According to Amelia Greenhall, there are two types of weight tracking: "I'm tracking to try and achieve a goal, or I'm tracking to try to maintain something—a level of activity or something that I'd like to continue." When tracking toward a set goal, for example losing 20 pounds, the day-to-day data gives you a lot of information and keeps you accountable to your goal. "But if you're just trying to maintain," said Greenhall, "just weighing yourself when you see the scale, and not worrying about getting on it every day, is a good enough measure."

Despite her personal preference to start with just a basic set of scales and a notepad, Greenhall does recognize the value of more advanced tools such as the Withings scale (which she herself now uses) and the Fitbit Aria scale. "They have a layer of design on them that is very accessible to mainstream," Greenhall reflected. She remarked that her mother and sister have started to use the Fitbit activity tracker scale. "They keep track of each other's steps and they've even brought my aunt in." However, she goes back to the issue of the day-to-day weight reading stressing people out. "One thing I would just love to see Withings scale do is just show you the trend number, not show you the real number. So it shows that your weight is going down, or the average of the last ten days." That's a big advantage of a scale being connected to the Internet, that it can calculate the trends on the fly. "Why can't they show you more friendly feedback than just this random number that you can get upset about?"

How Weight Watchers evolved to become a tracking system

Founder Jean Nidetch was the driving force in Weight Watchers for its first couple of decades. But in the 1990s the company realized that it needed to introduce a more rigorous scientific method into its programs. A support system and strict diet plans were no longer enough, especially since Weight Watchers now faced competition from a raft of science-based diets, from the low-carbohydrate Atkins diet to the low-fat diets then all the rage. The fact that many of those diets contradicted one another was beside the point. Weight Watchers needed to introduce its own science in order to compete.

Karen Miller-Kovach joined the company in 1993 as a registered dietitian. She's now the Chief Scientific Officer at Weight Watchers International and leads their research group. In the 2000s, Miller-Kovach became the official face of the company (not counting various celebrity endorsers, such as the actress Jennifer Hudson). With her blonde hair and trim—but not thin—figure, Miller-Kovach even closely resembled Jean Nidetch. Plus Miller-Kovach had a history of weight issues, just like her predecessor. Miller-Kovach told *USA Today* in 2005 that her weight problem had been caused by "a little too much of everything as opposed to too much of one thing." So if Nidetch couldn't control herself around cookies back in her self-described fat years, then it seems Miller-Kovach couldn't stop nibbling on lots of different foods. In a way, the eating problems of these two blonde Weight Watcher figureheads was mirrored in their differing philosophies for the company. Where Nidetch single-mindedly drove home the importance of set diets and a support system, Miller-Kovach couldn't help experimenting with a lot of new scientific formulas for Weight Watchers.

In the early days, calorie numbers weren't that important. The Weight Watchers formula of the 1960s and 70s was simple: follow this diet plan, to the letter, and you will lose weight. That's why the support system Nidetch pushed back then worked so well. The primary goal of Weight Watchers was to teach its members new eating habits. Nidetch understood that members would initially "cheat" on the diets, but over time the peer support system would win out and members would follow the plans strictly. "We help them develop self-control and self-respect," wrote Nidetch in her book *The Story of Weight Watchers*.

The set diet plans and support system worked very well, but by the 1980s Weight Watchers had decided to add some flexibility to its programs in order to attract new customers. So it introduced "exchange plans," enabling members to swap around (exchange) foods within a certain food category. For example, let's say you were allowed three servings of fruit per day. But if Monday's recommended breakfast featured half a cup of peaches and you didn't like peaches, then you could swap the peach for one small apple, or half a medium banana, or one cup of strawberries, or any other item on the exchange list. There was no breakdown of carbohydrates, protein or fat in any of these recommendations. It was mostly based on a single key measurement: calories. Half a cup of peaches roughly equaled one small orange in calories. But instead of letting its members obsess over the exact numbers of calories in each piece of fruit, Weight Watchers in the 1980s encouraged members to think of it in terms of the much simpler "exchanges." These food exchange lists weren't an innovation of Weight Watchers. The concept was popularized in the 1950s when an "exchange scheme" was promoted by the American Diabetes Association and the US Public Health Service to help diabetics keep track of their daily food intake.

When Weight Watchers introduced the food exchange lists in the 1980s, it not only added flexibility into its plans but it was also the company's first significant move into food tracking. However, with flexibility came more complexity. Especially since the Weight Watchers programs of the late 1980s, such as "The Quick Success Program," had different phases. There were typically five or six phases, which meant five or six different sets of menus.

The exchange lists were eventually replaced by a points system, introduced in 1997 under Miller-Kovach. This is when food tracking became the core of Weight Watchers. The new system allocated each food type a certain number of points based on calorie counts. For example, a large apple was allocated two points, a multi-grain English muffin one point, a Burger King bacon double cheeseburger twelve points and a glass of white wine two points. The point allocations were roughly the equivalent to calories—the apple was twice as calorie-heavy as the English muffin.

In effect, the Weight Watchers points were a greatly simplified system of calorie counting. How many points you had each day varied, but the average new member was allotted

22 daily points and an extra 35 weekly points. So that high-calorie Burger King burger? It would use up over half of your daily points, giving members a big incentive to avoid it.

In November 2010 Weight Watchers overhauled its points system and debuted an entirely new program called PointsPlus. The new system didn't just count calories, but also where those calories came from. Foods with high protein and fiber were assigned lower points, because they were seen by Weight Watchers as being a better form of calories. Meanwhile, foods high in fat and simple carbs were assigned higher values because they were viewed as being relatively bad calories. The idea was to encourage members to eat more of the high-protein and high-fiber products, and fewer of the high fat and high carb foods. Fresh fruits and non-starchy vegetables were taken off the points system altogether, meaning that members could eat as much of those foods as they liked.

Miller-Kovach said at the time PointsPlus was introduced that foods rich in protein and fiber "fill you up, keep hunger at bay, and help you lose weight in a healthier and more nutritious way." So the new system was essentially a more sophisticated form of calorie counting, taking into account recent trends in food science.

Under PointsPlus, most foods—other than fruit and non-starchy vegetables—had an increase in points. However, new members got a few more daily points to play with: 31 daily points (instead of 22) and 49 extra weekly points (instead of 35). The change in philosophy is best illustrated using the examples above. A large apple was now zero points, because all fruit was given a free rein. However, the English muffin had tripled from one to three points. Even though the muffin actually had fewer calories than the apple, the muffin attracted extra points because it was relatively high in fat. A glass of wine had doubled to four points. Interestingly though, the burger stayed the same at twelve points, making it now one-third of a member's daily points allotment, instead of a full half—one of the few consolations for junk-food eaters under the new system!

The new points formula was complicated, but that has been the gradual progression of Weight Watchers over the years: from over-simplified basic rules to complex formulas. The mastermind behind this shift, Karen Miller-Kovach, even claimed that the new PointsPlus system helped with behavior change. "In addition to weight loss," she said, "we found an improvement in behaviors that help people maintain weight loss and a reduction in the desire to eat when there's no physical hunger or need for food."

Is Weight Watchers institutionalized self-tracking? Yes, it can be thought of in those terms. Its points system is a sophisticated form of calorie counting, which makes it easy to track your food intake. You don't even need to attend face-to-face meetings in the Internet era of Weight Watchers. One of its programs, "Weight Watchers 360°," is an online self-tracking platform. It features online plan guides, a dashboard, and mobile apps similar to MyFitnessPal.

But 360° isn't the main offering of Weight Watchers. When it comes down to it, regardless of whether it's based on calories or exchanges or points, the support system anchors Weight Watchers. It's proven to be very helpful for people who either aren't as self-motivated as Amelia Greenhall, or who simply crave the companionship of fellow dieters.

Self-tracking for self-reflection

If America is going to tackle its problem with weight— remember that a third of the population are obese and a further third are overweight, according to WHO figures—its citizens first need to take more personal responsibility for their health. Tens of thousands of people already have, which is why Weight Watchers has been such an astounding success over the years. But there's so much more that can be done.

For people who want to lose weight and need structure and support, a commercial program like Weight Watchers is a good place to start. But there is an alternative and it's not that difficult. All you need is scales, a pen and notepad, and within a few weeks a spreadsheet. Amelia Greenhall has tracked her weight in this manner since 2007. The most important thing to do when self-tracking like Greenhall is to take a relaxed approach. She doesn't weigh herself every day and she focuses on the ten-day running average so that she doesn't become stressed about the daily fluctuations that always occur with weight. She also isn't concerned if she goes a month or two—or more—without weighing herself at all. If she is traveling or out in the woods hiking, she isn't weighing herself. But that's OK, because when she gets back she can resume her tracking and immediately see how her current weight compares to past patterns.

Tracking her weight has made Greenhall more aware of the role of diet in her wellbeing. She became a vegetarian about the same time that she began self-tracking, although she insists that it's not so much the type of diet she eats, but the fact that she now understands the impacts of certain foods on her body through tracking her weight over time. "I learned how to eat and how to cook," she explained. "That makes my body very happy. Just knowing what's really food and seeing that reflected in my body."

The overwhelming cause of the obesity epidemic in America and other Western countries is the poor food choices we make, given the relatively sedentary lives we lead. In the previous chapter we learned that by tracking the food we eat, we become more adept at choosing healthier foods. Likewise, by tracking your weight in the way that Amelia Greenhall does, you can see the effect of your food choices on your body.

But it's not just about the food. Self-tracking has also helped Greenhall find complementary activities that helped her lose and then maintain her weight. That's something I think Weight Watchers can learn from Greenhall and the self-tracking revolution: just as important as what you eat is finding activities that complement your lifestyle. That balance of proper eating and fun daily activity is key to weight maintenance. Since starting to track her weight in 2007, Amelia Greenhall has been able to see the benefits of biking from her weight spreadsheet: the more she biked, the better her weight. Perhaps that's an obvious correlation, but you'd be surprised how motivating it is to see that data on paper (or a computer screen).

The big difference between Amelia Greenhall's self-tracking approach to losing weight and that of Weight Watchers is in the source of motivation. With Weight Watchers, the motivation to keep going with weight control comes from peer support. But many people find that difficult to maintain, because the enjoyment factor isn't necessarily there, whereas self-tracking encourages you to be more self-aware and to find enjoyable ways to lose or maintain weight.

Like Amelia Greenhall, you can think of self-tracking as a form of self-reflection—similar to keeping a diary about your thoughts and feelings. Only with self-tracking for weight, the diary is about your body—about your weight patterns over time, what works in losing or maintaining weight, what you enjoy doing. Greenhall found that tracking her weight over time led to increased mindfulness about herself. She learned to treat herself better and not focus on numbers (or points, for that matter). Quite simply, self-tracking taught Amelia Greenhall to feel happy in her own skin.

CHAPTER FIVE

HOW USEFUL IS GENETICS? ME & MY 23ANDME RESULTS

Genomic information in a vacuum isn't all that useful yet, regardless of how low the cost.

Linda Avey, co-founder of 23andMe

On Monday November 19, 2007, my doctor told me I had type 1 diabetes. Coincidentally, November 19, 2007, was also the date that 23andMe launched its personal genetics service. Partly funded by Google, 23andMe was selling a DNA test direct to consumers for $1,000. The cost was high, but in return 23andMe promised its customers "deeper insights into their ancestry and other inherited traits which are marked in an individual's genetic code."

In hindsight, November 2007 was a watershed month, not just for me as a new diabetic, but for the consumer genomics industry. No fewer than three companies launched direct-to-consumer DNA tests in November 2007: 23andMe, deCODE genetics, and Navigenics. For the first time, ordinary people would be able to get their DNA tested without requiring a prescription from their doctor. Despite the high pricing from all three companies, there was a lot of interest in genetics at that time. The human genome had been fully sequenced just six years prior and there was no shortage of hype in the media about the potential medical benefits. Indeed, each of the three startups that launched in November 2007 was banking on that hype becoming reality. If genetics was going to lead to breakthroughs in disease prevention and maybe even cures, which was the common belief at the time, then there was a lot of money to be made in DNA tests.

When I discovered I had type 1 diabetes in November 2007 I didn't realize immediately that the disease had a genetic component, especially since I had no known family history of diabetes. Frankly, it was a huge shock to get the diagnosis. Type 1 (sometimes called juvenile diabetes) typically occurs in children, not adults. I'd recently turned 36, so it seemed to make no sense to me. It wasn't until nearly five years later, in September 2012, that I finally did a 23andMe DNA test. It was then I found out that I had a small genetic predisposition for type 1 diabetes.

I'd been aware of 23andMe since November 2007 (although the coincidence of its launch and my diagnosis occurring at the same time hadn't occurred to me till I began writing this chapter). So why did it take me so long to do the test? Partly it was the cost, which started off at $1,000 and didn't significantly drop until 2012. Partly it was that I'd had a health scare and it took me a long time to adjust. But mostly it was that I wasn't sure I wanted any more health surprises!

If the human genome was all the talk in the scientific and medical communities at the start of this century, then 23andMe was the best-placed Silicon Valley startup to attract attention in this developing field. It was the best funded, with a $9 million initial investment in May 2007. But it also helped that 23andMe co-founder and CEO Anne Wojcicki was one half of what passed as a celebrity couple in Silicon Valley. Her other half was Google co-founder Sergey Brin. Indeed, Google was one of the early investors in 23andMe, so the personal genomics venture had both nature (co-founded by a Silicon Valley insider) and nurture (funding from Google and other big hitters) to give it the right kind of start. Sure enough, in a classic case of survival of the fittest, 23andMe went on to become the dominant player in personal genomics, although that was helped by its two main competitors dropping out of the market—both deCODE Genetics and Navigenics were acquired and their direct-to-consumer businesses immediately shut down. Yet despite now having a virtual monopoly, 23andMe has dropped its price dramatically since 2007. At time of writing, it retails at under $100, less than a tenth of its original price.

Here's how 23andMe works. After you stump up the cash, you're sent a kit containing a plastic test tube. You spit into the test tube (the cells in your spit contain your DNA) and then return it to 23andMe. The company analyzes your spit in a process called "genotyping." It's important to point out that genotyping does not mean reading your entire genome. That would require 23andMe to read about three billion letters of your DNA, the unique combination of As, Ts, Gs, and Cs that make up your DNA codebase. Instead, 23andMe analyzes about one million letters of your DNA, which is not even 1% of your total DNA code.

Why does 23andMe only read such a small portion of your DNA? It's because most of the three billion letters in human DNA are the same from person to person. According to 23andMe, there are only about ten million places in the genome "where a single letter of the sequence sometimes differs from one person to the next." Those "one-letter spelling variations" are called SNPs, or single nucleotide polymorphisms. The SNPs (people in the industry pronounce them "snips") are what 23andMe analyzes, in particular the most information-rich one million of them.

My 23andMe results

Getting a genetics test isn't like most of the other forms of self-tracking we're exploring in this book. Your DNA doesn't change over time, so you only need to get the test done once. The main value of doing a genetics test, other than giving you information about your ancestry, is that it will identify risk factors for various diseases. In my case, my 23andMe results did indeed show that I had a higher than average chance of getting type 1 diabetes. According to 23andMe, I had a 4.1% risk of getting the disease during the course of my life. That's four times the average risk for men of European ethnicity. But 4.1% is still low, so there had to be other factors that triggered the disease in my body. More on that shortly. But for now let's focus on the genetics.

How did 23andMe come up with that 4.1% risk figure? The main factor, according to 23andMe, is an SNP labeled rs9273363. For the sake of easy recall, let's call this SNP Roger. Here is where we first encounter the problems of understanding genetics. It turns out that Roger isn't listed in the official online encyclopedia of SNPs, SNPedia. When I searched SNPedia, an excellent resource of SNP information, I found more than twenty SNPs known to be associated with type 1 diabetes. All of those SNPs were sourced from medical studies. But oddly, Roger wasn't one of them. However, a neighboring SNP is among the twenty, one labeled rs9272346. Let's call this SNP Peter. 23andMe also references Peter, but rejects it as "unreliable." 23andMe doesn't point to any evidence showing why Peter is unreliable—it just is, apparently. So what 23andMe does is swap the unreliable Peter for an SNP it deems more trustworthy: Roger. Both SNPs are on the same chromosome (6) and are closely positioned to each other. According to 23andMe, that means Roger "is also highly associated with type 1 diabetes."

At first I was confused about why 23andMe would cite a seemingly obscure SNP as its primary risk factor for type 1 diabetes. But on closer inspection I saw that 23andMe relies on the same major study that SNPedia cites. This study was published in *Nature* magazine in June 2007 by a group called The Wellcome Trust Case Control Consortium (WTCCC). According to its website, the WTCCC is a group of 50 research groups across the UK, established in 2005. The SNP referenced in SNPedia, Peter, is identified in the study as being associated with type 1 diabetes. The SNP that 23andMe uses, Roger, is not mentioned in the Wellcome study—which is why it didn't make it to SNPedia. But 23andMe is claiming that because they are such close neighbors in the genome, Peter and Roger are both markers for type 1 diabetes. I'll have to take their word for it, since 23andMe doesn't provide supporting evidence for this conclusion.

For the SNP that 23andMe used, rs9273363/Roger, my "genotype" was AA. A genotype is two letters (the A, T, G, or C of DNA code), one from your mother and the other from your father. An AA genotype for this gene has a relatively high risk factor for type 1 diabetes: 5.14 times the average risk (again, though, 23andMe doesn't explain how it came up with that figure). So Roger was the primary indicator used, but 23andMe also surveyed seven other SNP markers for type 1 diabetes. Peter wasn't among them. Of those seven SNPs, I had a slightly higher than average risk for three markers (but no more than 1.16% higher), and a slightly lower risk for four markers. Really, there was nothing among those other seven markers that jumped out. Overall, the other seven markers brought my risk *down* to 4.1%. So 23andMe is telling me that the genetic cause of my getting type 1 diabetes is most likely to be that one SNP: the mysterious Roger.

So what about rs9272346/Peter, the SNP that 23andMe rejected as "unreliable"? What was my genotype for that? 23andMe didn't tell me on its website, but the information is in the raw data file—the one million lines of SNP analysis that 23andMe did on my spit sample. Rather than look through the 25 megabyte text file, I ran it through a software program called Promethease (easily found via Google). Promethease compares your raw 23andMe data to SNPedia, then lists out any risks it finds. It showed that my genotype for Peter is also AA. But I was surprised to read in Promethease that an AA genotype for Peter is found in approximately one-third of all people. So it's a very common genotype! Also, this SNP appears to have a lower risk factor associated with it than the one 23andMe uses. Peter raises your likelihood of getting type 1 diabetes from 0.04% to 0.75%. That's a big jump from the average risk, because an AA genotype has eighteen times more risk. But 0.75% is still less than a 1% chance of getting type 1 diabetes. So overall, an AA genotype for Peter appears to be much less of a risk factor than the substitute SNP that 23andMe used, Roger.

You're beginning to see the problems of tracking your DNA. The "results" of a 23andMe test turn out to be a list of probabilities, which have been calculated by 23andMe based on relatively few major medical studies. Some of those studies are years old. The study for SNPs and type 1 diabetes was done in 2007, over six years ago as I write this. Is there nothing more recent? What's more, even if there is research cited, it seems that 23andMe is quite willing to override it. More than twenty possible SNP markers have been identified for type 1 diabetes in past research, yet the one chosen as primary marker by 23andMe is not even mentioned in the major medical study that it cites as proof. So 23andMe has substituted a SNP in that study with another SNP; but is it a true substitute when it has a completely different risk factor?

Perhaps this kind of concern was part of the reason why, in November 2013, the FDA warned 23andMe that its marketing was in violation of the Federal Food, Drug and Cosmetic Act (the FD&C Act). The FDA thought that 23andMe's reports could potentially mislead people about their health risks. This rap on the knuckles forced 23andMe to withdraw "health-related genetic reports" from its offering. As of mid-2014, 23andMe only provides new customers with "ancestry-related genetic reports and uninterpreted raw genetic data."

> **There are more questions than answers in the results of a 23andMe DNA test.**

My own biggest concern with 23andMe results is that even if I do (allegedly) have a higher than average genetic predisposition toward type 1 diabetes, ultimately that knowledge isn't very useful. That's because there is no known prevention strategy for the disease. So even if I didn't have the disease now, being told that I have an increased risk factor wouldn't help me prevent it. The best advice 23andMe is able to give me is to "consider talking to a genetic counselor." Talk about passing the buck.

So when it comes down to it, there are more questions than answers in the results of a 23andMe DNA test. This is where a new startup called Curious could help.

Curious for answers

Created by one of three co-founders of 23andMe, Linda Avey, Curious is an online community where people can ask questions about their health. The tagline of Curious is "we've got questions," which is an understatement in the case of genetics. Avey says the mission of Curious is "to build a platform that helps identify answers through data."

Linda Avey was a co-founder of 23andMe in April 2006, along with Paul Cusenza and current CEO Anne Wojcicki. In September 2009, Avey left the company to establish a foundation for Alzheimer's disease called the "Brainstorm Research Foundation." Both Avey and her husband have an increased genetic risk for the disease. But she wanted to go beyond just the genetic data and add other data to the mix, specifically "phenotypes," which is complementary information to the genotypes 23andMe assess.

A phenotype is the physical manifestation of genes, which means how the genes develop or behave. To use a familiar computing analogy: if the genome is your body's code, then phenotypes are the output of that code. As an example, your hair color is a phenotype. The color of your hair is programmed in your genes, but the resulting head of hair is the phenotype. When it comes to recording phenotypic information, it's all down to observation. One of Linda Avey's goals with the Brainstorm Research Foundation was to collect a large amount of phenotypic information from Alzheimer's patients—not just to study their genes, but also to gather information about how the disease developed in people who have those genes. "That's the part I really want to innovate," she told *Bio-IT World* magazine in 2009. "How can you use existing social networks like Facebook to become a platform for collection in a very systematic way?"

Avey's plan with the Brainstorm Research Foundation was to merge phenotypic and genetic data. However, this was soon usurped by a larger, more commercial vision. "I found that trying to do what I wanted to accomplish was better placed in a startup," Linda Avey told me in August 2013. "And not just focused on Alzheimer's." That led to the formation of Curious, a startup that she co-founded with two other people.

Rather than focus on just one disease, Curious aims to collect data about all diseases through a crowdsourced Q&A format. The idea is that people enter questions about a certain aspect of their health and others contribute observations from their own lives. At time of writing, the website (wearecurio.us) isn't yet live. But a series of example questions scrolls continuously down the homepage. One is: "Do blood glucose or insulin levels correlate with long-term risk for Alzheimer's?" Your blood glucose level is a type of phenotype, termed a "Metabolic Phenotype." It's a measurable part of your body and therefore an expression of your genetic code. So when people answer that question on Curious, based on their own life experience, it's a phenotype. If that person gives permission to Curious, their phenotype can be correlated to their genotype results from 23andMe. That in itself doesn't answer the main question, which was whether there is a correlation to Alzheimer's. But if Curious gathers enough answers to that question from different people, they can begin to figure out if people with an increased genotypic risk of Alzheimer's also tend to have higher than average blood glucose levels.

Phenotypic data is a big part of Curious, but Linda Avey told me that it will gather other types of information too. "We'll be looking at sensors, environmental feeds, microbiome," she told me, "… anything that people want to assemble together to look for patterns."

Curious is a very ambitious startup, because it will need a lot of answers and it'll be messy data. It won't be black and white much of the time, which means the patterns will be difficult to decipher. But regardless of whether Linda Avey succeeds in her latest venture, there is a need for services that help people utilize their genetic data in their daily healthcare. Linda Avey is acutely aware that the company she co-founded in 2006, 23andMe, doesn't deliver enough insights about our day-to-day health. "Genomic information in a vacuum isn't all that useful yet, regardless of how low the cost," she told the blog bionicly.com in 2013. What's needed, she said, is "the combination of genomic profiles with patient data, which will enable discovery of common and rare variants associated with diseases/conditions/drug response."

While the world waits for Curious and other startups to provide guidance, some people with a lot of innate curiosity have carried out their own research into their genetic data. Paul Clarke is such a person, a self-described "layperson doing DIY research" into his genome; however, it should be noted that he's a scientifically trained layperson. By day Paul Clarke is an electronics design engineer for a UK company that makes energy-saving fans and motors. But Clarke believes that anybody with a DIY mindset can find out a lot of actionable information about their genetic makeup, things that can ultimately improve their health.

Clarke reached out to me by email to say that he'd gotten a lot of benefit from 23andMe. He has studied the genetic data of about two dozen people. "At least 75% of the time," he told me, "we can find significant opportunities for improvement— not just awareness of risk." He went so far as to say that in one quarter of the cases he'd studied, there were "major gains or resolution of unsolved problems."

One of the genomes that Paul Clarke studied was his own, where he found "four major defects." Clarke had been ill at the time, with a variety of symptoms including migraines, hypothyroidism, and depression. But after studying his 23andMe results, he was able to implement changes into his lifestyle. He says that led him to "finally regain my health, return to work and resume a more normal life." Clarke's approach to studying his genome was a simple one: look for big jumps in risk. "A big spike can mean some metabolic process is broken," he explained.

One of the four major genetic problems that Paul Clarke found in his 23andMe results was a 50% increased risk of suffering a heart attack. Thanks to 23andMe, he was able to pinpoint the cause of the risk to the SNP rs10757278. "I found this by looking on the 23andMe page for heart disease," Clarke said. "It showed up as a tall red band, next to a bunch of much more minor ones." However, as we saw with my own type 1 diabetes risk, just knowing the SNP involved and the risk factor isn't enough. "The thing is," said Clarke, "this defect is neither named nor understood. It's simply a case of statistical evidence based on millions of people's family history. People with a defect at that position have elevated risk." There was no indication in 23andMe about what this particular piece of DNA does. In fact rs10757278 has also been connected with other diseases: depression, fatigue, and dementia. But they're all just statistical associations. "In 23andMe it's just a red bar," Clarke told me. "You have to go looking to find more information."

The first thing Paul Clarke did was look at SNPs that were on the same chromosome and very near the one that 23andMe had identified, rs10757278. "My theory was that maybe the defect caused some kind of read error that disrupted stuff around it," explained Clarke. "I'd read of defects doing that, and it made sense." In other words, maybe it wasn't the SNP that 23andMe pinpointed that caused his increased risk of heart disease. Maybe that SNP caused nearby genes to malfunction. "What I found was interesting," continued Clarke. "It turns out that near this defect (rs10757278), in the 9p21 region, are three genes: one related to tumor suppression, one RNA gene that's not understood, and a gene that encodes a protein that converts scavenged sulfur into methionine." That third gene attracted Clarke's interest, because he had been having problems with anything that gave off fumes. Onions, garlic, leeks, and diesel exhaust would all make his heart pound and his face grow red—a symptom of heart problems. Sulfur was present in diesel exhaust, so was there a connection?

Clarke formulated a theory. Perhaps rs10757278 interfered with the gene responsible for his body's manufacture of methionine. If that theory turned out to be correct, that would explain his heart palpitations when exposed to fumes. He also discovered, through further research, that there had been cases of industrial sulfur poisoning causing congestive heart failure. It was all apparently connected. Yet he still hadn't proven anything. It could all be coincidence and his heart problems completely unrelated to sulfur.

The next step in his DIY research was to find out more about methionine, the hormone that he reasoned his body was having problems producing. "I looked up L-methionine deficiency and learned about the homocysteine cycle." He discovered that disruptions to the homocysteine cycle are definitely related to heart disease. Now he was onto something … "My next question," continued Clarke, "was, can I order L-methionine OTC from Amazon? Why yes!" Two days later the UPS truck arrived and Clarke gobbled down 500 mg of methionine, having looked up a typical dosage given in cases of deficiency. "The result was startling," he exclaimed. "Within fifteen minutes of taking L-methionine, I had a remarkable boost in mood, energy, and mental capacity."

L-methionine is an amino acid supplement that is available over the counter and, of course, on Amazon.com, but it's important to point out that it does have side effects. That was a concern for Paul Clarke because he had other health problems he was taking medication for—the hypothyroidism, for one. So he quickly informed his doctor about his L-methionine discovery. "She heard my theories and what I'd found, and confirmed it. It appeared I'd correctly worked it all out." But he added that she also provided a vital piece of support. "Now that my homocysteine cycle was working," his doctor explained to him, "I'd better start taking a multi-B vitamin supplement, because I'd be causing some new problems if I ran out of B vitamins! So that was a very useful addition to making sure my treatment was really healthy. That was not something I could have done by myself."

Paul Clarke's DIY research into his genetic data shows that sometimes the answer to a genetic defect is as simple as taking a supplement. However, it also shows the value of collaborating with your doctor in your findings.

It needn't be as serious a health problem as Paul Clarke suffered. Even genetic data that reveals just a small increased risk can be useful information to present to your doctor. Dr. Tim Janzen is a native Oregonian who has practiced medicine at South Tabor Family Physicians, Portland, since 1990. Dr. Janzen has a special interest in genealogy, from both a medical and an ancestry perspective. He's written guest blog posts for 23andMe about using DNA data to track his ancestors and is a member of the "23andMe Ancestry Ambassadors group." While Dr. Janzen's focus is mostly on the ancestry research applications of genetics data, he's also adamant about its benefits in preventative medicine. He commented in *Forbes* magazine:

> *I spend [a] significant part of my day telling my patients to 'eat right, don't smoke and get plenty of exercise.' Some follow my advice, but many don't. Perhaps at least a percentage of my non-compliant patients would be more motivated to change their behavior if they had genetic data that suggested they are at higher risk for heart disease, diabetes, and other conditions for which a healthy lifestyle would be helpful in reducing their overall risk.*

Taking your 23andMe results to your doctor can be a useful exercise because your doctor knows your medical history and can help you decipher some of your genetic risk factors. That said, using genetics for medical diagnosis is still very new to the scientific community. In short, there's a limit to what your

Using genetics for medical diagnosis is still very new to the scientific community.

doctor understands about genetics. Consider this factoid from Eric Vallabh Minikel, a computational scientist at the Center for Human Genetic Research at Massachusetts General Hospital in Boston. Of the fewer than one million SNPs that 23andMe genotypes, Minikel wrote in March 2013, "science can only offer confident and meaningful health interpretations [for] about 10,000 or 20,000 of them at most." The remaining SNPs, according to Minikel, cover ancestry, finding relatives, and "allow 23andMe's researchers to discover new trait associations in the future." That's not even counting the rest of the three billion letters in our DNA that 23andMe doesn't even read.

So, much is still unknown in both the scientific and medical professions about which genes are associated with diseases. If there is any one group of professionals who are most qualified to diagnose disease using genetics, it's probably those in the nascent field of "genetics counseling"—a specialized occupation that requires a master's degree. At the present time, genetics counselors typically focus on one of two areas of healthcare: prenatal and cancer counseling. According to a 2012 survey by the National Society of Genetic Counselors, over half of its 3,000 members work in one of those two specialties. Often genetics counselors do testing that goes much deeper than the genotyping offered by 23andMe. In a June 2013 article in the *Johns Hopkins Magazine*, Carolyn Applegate, a genetics counselor at the Institute of Genetic Medicine, commented that "whole-exome testing" has become popular in the profession. Such testing not only reads a person's genome, but "looks across all the protein coding parts of genes at once to see if we can find a change that would explain an individual's condition."

Genetics counseling may be helpful if you have a very serious health risk, such as cancer. But in most cases doing a 23andMe test and your own DIY research afterwards is probably your best strategy in using your DNA to help prevent disease.

Epigenetics: nature vs. nurture

So let's come back to this notion of disease prevention. That really is at the heart of 23andMe's genetic tests. Given knowledge of the risk factors for various diseases, we are better prepared to prevent those diseases. That's the theory that 23andMe is pushing anyway.

Paul Clarke's 23andMe results came back with what he termed "four major defects." I was lucky in comparison. My own 23andMe results revealed only one major health risk: type 1 diabetes. I also had a higher than average risk of getting melanoma, but that wasn't a surprise given my pale complexion. So overall I felt that the genetics gods were well disposed toward me—except for type 1 diabetes, which unfortunately I had acquired about five years before my 23andMe test. Of course, I have wondered whether knowing I had a predisposition toward that disease *before* I got it would have helped me prevent it.

Since 23andMe deals in probabilities, let's analyze the numbers it served up to me. As I noted earlier in this chapter, 4.1% was the magic number I was given—representing my risk of developing type 1 diabetes. Specifically, 23andMe informed me, "4.1 out of 100 men of European ethnicity who share Richard MacManus's genotype will develop type 1 diabetes between the ages of 0 and 79." The average is one out of 100 men of European ethnicity (1%). So I had a risk factor of over four times the average.

But 4.1% is a pretty low risk, even though it's four times the normal risk. It gets even lower when I adjust the age range in 23andMe's odds calculator. I was diagnosed with type 1 diabetes soon after I turned 36. According to 23andMe, "0.16 out of 100 men of European ethnicity who share Richard MacManus's genotype will develop type 1 diabetes between the ages of 30 and 39." So my genetic risk was *much* lower than 1% for getting type 1 diabetes in my thirties, which I did. OK, I still had a higher than average risk in the thirties age group, since the average was less than 0.1 out of 100. But still, a risk of just over one in a thousand is tiny odds.

With that in mind, there's an increasing school of thought that holds that genetics usually play a very small part in developing a disease, though there are certainly cases where genetics is the main contributing factor. For example, early-onset Alzheimer's disease is, in most cases, inherited through genes. But early-onset Alzheimer's disease is relatively rare, making up less than 5% of all people who have Alzheimer's. The more common form, nicknamed "late-onset" because it generally develops after age 60, is thought to be caused by a combination of genetic, environmental, and lifestyle factors.

So was it just bad luck that I got type 1 diabetes when I did? Given that the odds were 1/1000, you'd have to say it was. But it also strongly suggests that my environment had something to do with me getting this disease. Type 1 diabetes is an autoimmune disease, caused by the body's immune system attacking the insulin-producing cells of the pancreas. Essentially, the disease kills off your body's ability to produce insulin, meaning that type 1 diabetics need to inject insulin every day in order to survive. But nobody knows why the immune system attacks the pancreas in that way. There was a tiny genetic risk in my case, but clearly something triggered it in my body, something in my environment, which could mean anything from the foods I ate to the air I breathed.

Several environmental factors that *may* increase your risk of getting type 1 diabetes are listed by 23andMe, including "living in a cold climate, exposure to certain viruses, and not being breastfed as an infant." Those factors were all sourced from two medical studies, one a 1995 "population-based study of young Danish twins" and a 2003 study of "22,650 young Finnish twin pairs." Not only are those references over a decade old, but the studies also appear to have been quite small.

So back to my original question: could I have prevented the onset of type 1 diabetes, knowing my increased risk for it? Based on the very low genetic odds I had and the unknown environmental factors that eventually triggered the disease, then I have to say no, I couldn't have prevented it.

It all comes down to epigenetics, which is a recent trend in the field of genomics. Epigenetics literally means "control above genetics"—meaning, "control by the environment." However, it's not that the environment changes your genes; it's that the environment changes the *expression* of your genes. Your genes are contained in cells, and environmental factors cause changes at the cellular level, which in turn affect how your genes are expressed in your body.

We won't delve into the technicalities here, but there is one key insight from epigenetics that helped me come to terms with my 23andMe results. As virologist Nessa Carey put it in her book *The Epigenetics Revolution*, your DNA is like a script or a blueprint. "The same script is used differently depending on its cellular context," wrote Carey. Put another way, if I lived out my life 100 times, I would probably only develop type 1 diabetes a few times (well, four if I go by the 23andMe odds). That's because in 96 out of my 100 lifetimes, my environment would *not* cause changes in my cells that in turn trigger the disease.

In a nutshell, epigenetics is where nature meets nurture. The problem is that there are many things in our nurture that we have no direct control over. A virulent flu virus, for example, would be very difficult to avoid, unless you locked yourself away from society for the duration of the epidemic (an unknown virus is one of the leading "smoking gun" suspects for triggering type 1). You also can't control your early years, not only as a baby but also as a fetus. Whether you were breastfed is apparently one of the possible links to type 1 diabetes. But if a mother is malnourished when she is pregnant, that can also cause cellular changes in her fetus—in other words, epigenetic changes that could cause disease in the future life of her child.

The main aspect of nurture that you can control here and now, to a certain degree at least, is what you put into your body: what you eat and drink. Nutrition is in fact a key area in the study of epigenetics. In her book, Nessa Carey gives the example of how taking the supplement folic acid in the early stage of pregnancy helps reduce the baby's chances of developing spina bifida. But Carey warns that applying epigenetics to nutrition is speculative at this time. It's the same problem I outlined earlier regarding 23andMe results. The scientific community doesn't yet know precisely how certain foods, for example, affect the expression of our genes. Our bodies are enormously complex, because we have three billion genes and they all interact with each other, *and* with the environment, hormones in the body, and so forth.

Should you do a 23andMe test?

This raises the following question: how useful is a 23andMe test when so much about genetics is still unknown, and when the environment probably plays a much bigger role in triggering disease anyway?

As we've seen in this chapter, 23andMe results are all based on statistical probabilities. Often the studies they're based on are small (a sample of 1,000–2,000 people) and from faraway countries like Norway and Sweden. Some of these reports are five, ten, or more years old. Overall, the scientific community has been able to find a direct correlation between genes and diseases in far less than 1% of all genes. That's incredibly low and just shows how little we know about genetics at this stage of human evolution. Also, we've seen in recent years how the environment has become a more prominent factor in the way the scientific community thinks about health and disease. The study of epigenetics shows that everything from what your mother ate in the early stages of her pregnancy, to what you eat now, can cause cellular changes that may trigger certain diseases. But again, we know very, very little about what specifically in our foods or environment causes those changes.

All of this sparse evidence suggests that genetics tests are not very useful at this time. However, from a holistic point of view I'm still very glad I got a 23andMe test. OK, it didn't change the fact that I got type 1 diabetes. I had a very small genetic predisposition, but there was nothing I could have done to prevent it. Nevertheless, my 23andMe results did give me more knowledge about the makeup of my body. Despite my body still being very much a black box—much of its data locked up inside of me, unknowable or indecipherable at this time—I'm comforted that my self-knowledge has increased, even by just a percentage point or two.

As Paul Clarke showed, knowing more about your genetic makeup enables you to at least try to track down the cause of any future illness, or try to improve an aspect of yourself, through what science has discovered about certain SNPs to date. I feel better knowing that I can do my own research, based on my 23andMe data. And 23andMe also gives you information about yourself that is useful when monitoring your health over time. If you have an above-average risk of getting heart disease, then you may want to get regular cholesterol tests. You know what to watch out for.

I was pleased enough with my own 23andMe results that I offered to buy the test for members of my family. Their differing responses are a good indication of society's comfort level with genetic testing at this time. My parents, in their mid-sixties, politely declined my offer. My mother and father decided that they would rather not know at this time in their lives. Fair enough, I thought. I have three siblings and two took me up on the offer. My sister, the youngest of my family, took the test and shared her results with me on the 23andMe website. One of my brothers declined to take up my offer. The other accepted it, but when the test kit arrived from 23andMe he demurred. Soon after he received the kit, there was a newspaper article in New Zealand stating there is a legal obligation to declare to health insurance companies that you have done a genetics test. I can understand my brother's hesitation, because it's quite clear that in my country there is a risk of being declined coverage if his genetics test throws up a curveball. The US thankfully doesn't have that risk. The Genetic Information Nondiscrimination Act of 2008 prevents discrimination in insurance or employment based on genetic test results.

Quite apart from insurance concerns, you need to ask yourself whether you're prepared for the potentially bad news that 23andMe could deliver. And 23andMe itself is sensitive to this, as by default two of the health risk reports it delivers are locked: for Alzheimer's disease and Parkinson's disease. That's because you cannot do much to prevent those diseases, even if you have an increased risk. So you have to choose to manually unlock those reports, if you wish to know. In an almost cavalier manner, I chose to view them. Thankfully, I had a typical or decreased risk for both Alzheimer's and Parkinson's. But looking back on that, I wonder whether I had the mental strength at the time to deal with an enhanced risk factor for either disease. I already had type 1 diabetes, so I was worried enough about my health as it was. Would the additional risk factor have caused too much stress for my body to handle?

As with all the forms of tracking covered in other chapters in this book, ultimately it comes down to a personal choice.

The 23andMe test results come with many more questions than answers. Some of those questions are deeply personal ones. Can you handle the truth? Will it potentially prevent you from getting health insurance? And so on. Only you can answer those questions for your own circumstances.

The good news, however, is that knowing more about your genetic makeup can help you as a self-tracker. It alerts you to things about your body to keep an eye on. And maybe, just maybe, your 23andMe results will one day be the key to solving a future health problem.

CHAPTER SIX

INCEPTION: TRACKING THE BRAIN

I don't see the focus as neuroscience. It's helping people become more self-aware, and neuroscience is just one channel through which you can do that.

Crystal Goh, co-founder of Neuroprofile

Crystal Goh is a 26-year-old neuroscientist. A native of Hong Kong, but with a strong American accent, Goh is in the final stages of her PhD at Berkeley. She has also started a company on the side, with the intention of devoting herself fully to it after she graduates. The nascent company, called Neuroprofile, is focused on the human brain. It's an ambitious project that aims to help people track changes in their brain activity through MRI imaging. The method may sound lofty—maybe even a bit scary—but the goal is straightforward. Crystal Goh wants to show people the strengths and weaknesses in their brain so they know what they need to work on.

I met up with Crystal in January 2013 at a popular student café on the Berkeley campus, called Caffe Strada. It was a fine crisp winter's morning and we sat outside on the patio, underneath a healthy-looking pear tree. Yellow leaves from the tree drifted down onto our table as we talked. The café was full, both inside and out. Some tables were occupied by lone students with tousled hair, heads down, scribbling in notebooks or peering into MacBook screens. Other tables had couples or groups of students, all engaged in happy, earnest chatter. Every now and then an attractive young person would jog past on the sidewalk, as full of vitality as the yellow flowering pear trees. With all this youth and vigor around me, I almost felt like a student again myself.

Small of stature, Crystal had long, jet-black hair and was wearing a dark brown faux fur scarf to ward off any lingering winter bitterness—of which there seemed little chance in this part of the San Francisco Bay Area. She had sharp, penetrating eyes (I wondered, is she trying to read my mind?). But there was a warmth about her, too. She was talkative, as if energized by the sunny, youthful surroundings. We got to know each other by chatting about Eastern philosophy, Crystal sipping a chai tea and me a light, frothy cappuccino. I wondered how many of the shiny groups of students in this café were also talking about theology. Ah, to be young again and a Berkeley student, I sighed inwardly. But I snapped out of this fanciful daydream when Crystal began to tell me about the evolution of her startup.

Inception

After studying psychology at the University of Bristol in England in 2010, Goh earned a scholarship to do her PhD at University College London. But she was in two minds about what to specialize in. "I had two weeks to decide what I wanted to do with it," she told me. "I happened to watch *Inception* that week, and," she chuckled, "I was like, alright, I'm gonna do some sleep research."

Inception is a 2010 science-fiction film written and directed by Christopher Nolan, who went on to direct the latest franchise of Batman films. Nolan's script was inspired by lucid dreaming—a state of mind in which you're dreaming, but you're consciously aware of it. Technically, lucid dreaming is a brain phenomenon caused by an increased level of activity in the parietal lobes. In the movie, Leonardo DiCaprio plays Dominic Cobb, a corporate espionage thief who infiltrates the subconscious of his victims while they're asleep and dreaming, and extracts information. When caught, he's offered a chance to regain his freedom if he successfully completes a task considered to be impossible: "inception," the implanting of an idea into someone's subconscious, in other words, altering the thoughts inside a person's brain. This elaborate plot, which I recall was almost impossible to follow, inspired Crystal Goh to study sleep and dreams for her PhD.

After a couple of years studying sleep, brain imaging, and "non-invasive brain stimulation" at University College in London, she crossed the Atlantic to complete her PhD at Berkeley's Sleep and Neuroimaging Lab. At the lab, she is helping conduct a study of how sleep deprivation impacts self-awareness.

Even though she's a full-time student, Goh has already co-founded a startup in order to capitalize on her neuroscience skill-set. Called Neuroprofile, the consumer side of it will offer brain imaging and interpretation to everyday people. Unlike the plot of *Inception*, Goh's goal

> "You can understand yourself by tracking changes in your brain."

with Neuroprofile is to simplify the act of brain imaging. "What we want to do is simply show people their brains," she said. The idea is to identify parts of the brain that need improvement.

Goh insisted that there is nothing "that special" about seeing a visualization of your brain. "Once you demystify it," she said of the human brain, "and see what kind of data it contains, then it becomes another reflection of yourself." She compared getting regular MRIs of your brain to counting your steps with a Fitbit: "You can understand yourself by tracking changes in your brain."

How Neuroprofile will work

Neuroprofile currently has three components: a consumer service, software for clinicians, and an academic service.

The consumer service will enable people to order an expert analysis of their brain image. However, there are a number of obstacles to this plan. For a start, Neuroprofile won't help people actually get an MRI scan—although it hopes to partner with scanning centers in future. For now the user will need to schedule an MRI scan independently, get a digital copy of the result, and upload that to Neuroprofile. The trouble is, getting an MRI is not like going to the dentist. You can't simply walk off the street into an MRI center and request a brain scan. You're only likely to get a brain MRI if your doctor orders it for a medical reason, or you end up in the hospital with a head injury. What's more, even if you get an MRI scan, it's questionable whether you can get a digital copy of it. That's especially problematic in the US, where there is strict security around medical imaging. "We're still working out who actually owns it," said Goh of MRI scans in the US. "Whether it's the patient, the scanner, or the insurance company who owns it here … or maybe nobody does."

Because of the practical issues in the US, Neuroprofile will use Europe as its testing ground. That's because Europe is more open to consumers having access to their digital MRI scans. "In the UK, there's something called the Data Protection Act," explained Goh. "Which means that you have the right to your own raw data."

For their first customers, Goh said that Neuroprofile will target university experiments in Europe—particularly in London. It also aims to appeal to so-called citizen scientists, people who contribute to scientific research via the Internet. "What we want to encourage people to do is participate in an fMRI experiment," said Goh. "The 'f' in fMRI stands for functional," she added, "which is a scan of your brain's blood oxygen level." Participants in these university experiments will "almost always" get a structural scan as well, according to Goh. A structural MRI scan looks at the anatomical structure of the brain. From these two types of MRI scan, functional and structural, Goh says that Neuroprofile will be able to provide a useful analysis of the brain.

So what kind of information will you learn from Neuroprofile, provided you've jumped through all the hoops and uploaded your MRI scan into the service? First, your brain will be compared to a baseline of other brains. The baseline will ideally be the brains of other people of the same sex, similar age and background, along with other optional factors, such as educational background and even IQ score. The Neuroprofile software then looks for differences between your own brain and the chosen baseline. Those differences become the focus for potential self-improvement.

Like most of the startup founders profiled in this book, Goh has been using herself as the initial test subject for her product. "What I found was that my tool-handling area was significantly lower in gray matter density, compared to 200 other people." Goh explained that tool-handling in this context means "an area of the brain that is not solely responsible for tool use, but is consistently involved in experiments where we ask people to handle tools." So it would be expected that, say, a carpenter would have a high gray matter density in this region of the brain.

Knowing your tool-handling ability may or may not be useful information to you. While it may explain why you're not good at DIY projects around the house, is it something you necessarily want to focus your energies on improving? Probably not. All of us have specific skills and we've honed them through many, many hours of use. The more you do something, the better at it you get. Malcolm Gladwell's "10,000-Hour Rule" comes to mind. In his book *Outliers: The Story of Success*, Gladwell wrote that "ten thousand hours of hard practice" is a key factor in very successful people. So an MRI will likely highlight areas of your brain that you already know you're good at, because you do it a lot. Vice versa for areas of your brain you don't use as much. This is all interesting data to know, but won't propel you to make lifestyle changes.

However, other parts of your brain may be more important to you. In Crystal Goh's case, she identified emotion regulation as something in her brain that she'd like to improve. At a presentation to the Silicon Valley Quantified Self Meetup, in December 2012, Goh explained how her brain scan revealed that the part of her brain responsible for emotional regulation was lower in gray matter density than other brains. Since that scan, she has increased her sitting meditation and daily sleep hours. She reasons that these lifestyle changes will help improve her emotional regulation. She plans to check whether it has or not, in her next scan.

Changing your mind

You may be asking, Is it really that easy to alter my own brain? Well, yes, in many ways the brain can actually change. The technical term for this is "neuroplasticity." Also known as cortical re-mapping, it refers to the brain's ability to reorganize itself by forming new neural connections. That's essentially what Goh is attempting to do to the emotional regulation area of her brain by meditating and sleeping more.

Neuroplasticity is a fancy word, but Goh insists it's not as difficult as it sounds. The Neuroprofile website states that neuroplasticity "is not so complicated, it's simply a matter of changing behavioral patterns." And change is a key part of Crystal Goh's goal with Neuroprofile. "I care a lot about making and instilling change in people's lives," she told me. "The brain is a mere proxy of health and wellness, so there are things to navigate." Over time, Goh wants to partner with specialists to help people implement any behavioral change that their brain scans recommend. "My dream is to work with nutritionists, neurologists, therapists, life coaches, Chinese medicine doctors … basically anyone who can teach us how to live better and healthier."

Many behavioral patterns in your brain can be changed by making lifestyle changes or doing exercises to train the brain— for example, visual exercises to improve your visual processing ability. But sometimes your brain needs what Crystal Goh termed "brain stimulation," in other words, an electric current applied to your head. I raised my eyebrows at that and told Goh that the thought of someone tampering with my brain scared me. She tried to reassure me. "Oh, it's not scary at all. It's very low voltage. So, you're talking about, like, one milliamp." My eyebrows remained raised, so Goh explained further. "All you're doing is ..." she said, searching for a way to put this in layman's terms. But she gave up and decided to tell it to me straight. "So, your brain fires because there are electrical potentials. By injecting a current, you're lowering the potential, so it fires more easily. That's it."

I nodded, but in the back of my brain I was still thinking about all those horror stories of electric shock therapy I'd read about in the past. New Zealand novelist Janet Frame, American rock legend Lou Reed, the popular Brazilian writer Paolo Coelho. All had suffered this horrific so-called therapy. Nowadays, electric shock treatment is known as "electroconvulsive therapy" (ECT) and, remarkably, it's still widely used as a treatment for severe depression. And that's the kind of mind association that Crystal Goh and her business partners will have to contend with when marketing to prospective customers. The brain stimulation that Goh refers to is, medically speaking, a totally safe procedure. But even so, I'm not sure I'd be willing to do it. I've filed brain stimulation away, in my mind, as something akin to laser treatment for nearsightedness. Sure, it may be an entirely safe procedure and even a good idea, but there's no way I'm letting a laser near my eyes. Likewise, the thought of electricity being applied to my brain is off-putting.

So customer fear, whether justified or not, is another challenge Crystal Goh will have to overcome with Neuroprofile. But she is determined to brush aside these obstacles. Indeed, she points to Japan as a country that already has routine brain scanning clinics.

Brain docks

In Japan there is a common brain check-up procedure known as a "brain dock." The first brain dock appeared in 1988 at the Sapporo neurosurgery hospital. In 1992, an official organization for brain docks, the Japan Brain Dock Society, was founded.

According to Dr. T. Ohta, a clinical neurosurgeon at the Institute of Brain Function, Iseikai Hospital in Osaka, a brain dock is a special clinic where people go to get their brain scanned. This is done in order to detect brain diseases. In a chapter for a 2006 book entitled *Medical Technologies in Neurosurgery*, Dr. Ohta wrote that "such brain dock clinics are very popular in Japan, while they have rarely been reported from abroad." Dr. Ohta went on to explain that it costs about US$500 to attend such a clinic. Despite the high price, brain docks are used by many Japanese people, in particular the elderly, who are worried about the impact of mental or physical diseases on "their family's happiness and harmony."

The brain dock was inspired by a broader medical checkup commonly performed in Japan, known as the "ningen dock." Over one or two days, a patient undergoes a series of medical tests and X-rays. They also have a consultation with a doctor to talk about their medical history and lifestyle habits. Dr. Minoru Yamakado, from the Japan Society of Ningen Dock, details what happens next:

> Later that day, after the exams have finished,
> the doctor explains the results to the client in an
> interview, and gives lifestyle advice on how the client
> can maintain their health. One feature of the ningen
> dock is that it emphasizes both the consultation and
> the post-examination interview.

The ningen dock has a long history, dating back to 1954, when it was a six-day health check-up. The word "ningen" means "human." The term "ningen dock" was coined by the Japanese newspaper *Yomiuri Shimbun*, which compared the process to the maintenance a ship undergoes after a sea voyage. The ningen dock in contemporary Japanese society is "an essential part of the way that Japanese people maintain their health," according to Dr. Yamakado. He wrote that about three million people receive the ningen dock every year, at 1,500 medical institutions around the country. While the brain dock isn't as prevalent, it's the same principle of regularly monitoring (at a "dock") one's health.

This type of monitoring and analysis is exactly what all the health technology products profiled in this book aim to do, in one form or another. Data from your Fitbit device is uploaded to the Internet, where you can analyze it on the Fitbit website. Likewise, Crystal Goh's Neuroprofile scans your brain and will help you make improvements to your cognitive abilities. So, in a sense, Japan pioneered the very same concepts of self-awareness and health tracking that consumer web startups like Fitbit and Neuroprofile are implementing now; in addition, the 10,000 steps per day metric that Fitbit uses as its baseline for an "active" lifestyle came from a Japanese pedometer company in the 1970s.

Given all this, I wasn't surprised to learn that Japan is a key market for Goh, and her two business partners, and co-founders, are Japanese. Yoshinobu Kano is a machine learning expert in Japan, while Dr. Ryota Kanai is a former colleague of Goh's from the Institute of Cognitive Neuroscience in London. "Japan is really progressive," Goh said, citing the brain docks. "It's common for people to get a brain scan as a preventative measure."

Other than selling brain scans direct to consumers, Neuroprofile also plans to make money by licensing its software technology to clinicians. Goh sees the technology as being useful to hospitals and medical clinics. Currently, clinicians in the Japanese brain docks scan MRI images primarily to look for brain disease. But Goh wants to enable Japanese brain clinicians to do "more research-based" activities as well, such as "machine learning algorithms to help predict, for example, Alzheimer's onset," which in turn could help people at risk of developing Alzheimer's to implement prevention methods much earlier. "If you can predict Alzheimer's three years before it kicks in," explained Goh, "then early intervention may curb your cognitive impairment."

Crystal's yin and yang brain

This was a lot of new information for my own brain to handle. I sat back and rested my pen on the table beside my notebook, then smiled and scratched my forehead. Her penetrating eyes remained fixed on me. Perhaps it was all this talk of future potential for brain scans. While it appeared to have leverage in Japan, it's more like science fiction in the US. To try to bridge the gap, I asked Crystal Goh how, with her Hong Kong upbringing and Eastern philosophical sensibilities, she ended up at one of the most famous universities in America?

Goh told me that she was born and raised in Hong Kong, but her background is a mix of Eastern and Western influences. The American accent I detected at the start of our interview comes in part from attending the Chinese International School, a private school in Hong Kong that has many international teachers. Her parents were Methodists, a very Western religion, but at the age of sixteen she became fascinated by yoga and meditation.

She was also steeped in the health world from an early age, with both her parents being doctors. Her mother is a radiologist, and Goh remembers looking at lots of X-rays and MRI scans when she was growing up. But as has been the case for millions of teenagers the world over, Goh's first career goal was diametrically opposed to what her parents did for a living. "I never wanted to be in this field. I was going to be an artist actually." So she went to art school in 2005, in London. But, subconsciously, the medical field had an irresistible pull for her. For one art project, she wanted to use an endoscope and make a video of it going through a person's body. When that project failed to interest her art teachers, she decided to quit art school, and in 2006 she began studies at a medical school in Bristol. She changed her mind again shortly after. "After the first week, I switched to psychology." This got her on the track of neuroscience. "I got exposed to neuroscience and I discovered there was a lot that wasn't understood about the brain. It was the last frontier of the human body that needed to be thoroughly understood. I felt like it was really important."

As she continued her study of the brain, Goh began to realize that her Eastern background and teenage fascination with meditation overlapped with her field of study. She started thinking about how neuroscience could help people become more mindful of their bodies and lifestyles. "I don't see the focus of what I do as neuroscience," she told me. "I see the focus as helping people become more self-aware, and neuroscience is just one channel through which you can do that. You can meditate, you can read books, you can go on a retreat. There are many different ways. You can track yourself with Fitbit. Neuroscience happens to be what I specialize in."

Goh sees Eastern philosophies, and practices like meditation and yoga, as being as useful for self-examination and awareness as the technical tools of the West. Indeed, she recently started meditating again in the Zen manner. "I think Eastern and Western interventions should be used together," she mused. "Why not? We have all those tools."

"I think Eastern and Western interventions should be used together."

There are in fact scientific studies proving that meditation physically changes, and improves, the brain. In a study published in the January 2011 edition of the journal *Psychiatry Research: Neuroimaging*, researchers found that just eight weeks of daily meditation is enough to change brain structure. There were sixteen "healthy, meditation-naïve" participants in the study, who practiced meditation for an average of 27 minutes per day over eight weeks. Each participant got an MRI of their brain before the study started and another MRI eight weeks later. The second MRI showed significant changes in the areas of the brain associated with learning, memory, and regulation of emotions. According to a report in the *Harvard Gazette*, the study found "increased gray-matter density in the hippocampus, known to be important for learning and memory, and in structures associated with self-awareness, compassion, and introspection." The researchers also found "decreased gray-matter density in the amygdala, which is known to play an important role in anxiety and stress." Britta Hölzel, a research fellow at Massachusetts General Hospital and Giessen University in Germany, was the first author of the study. She told the *Harvard Gazette*, "It is fascinating to see the brain's plasticity and [to see that] that, by practicing meditation, we can play an active role in changing the brain and can increase our wellbeing and quality of life."

Ultimately, Crystal Goh is trying to use the physiology of the brain to help us understand our bodies and lifestyles. The intermingling of Western and Eastern brain "interventions"— shots of electrical currents are the yin and meditation the yang—is the path to self-improvement in Goh's world.

So what brought Crystal Goh to Berkeley and Silicon Valley? In many ways it goes back to the philosophical questions her teenage self grappled with. She recalls going through some personal issues as a teenager (as we all do during that time of our lives) and constantly examining herself. "Why am I feeling this? What is the root of this? Is it chemicals in my brain? Is it some mystical force that I don't know?"

These were some of the electrical thoughts that zipped through Crystal Goh's teenage mind. Nowadays, she's tackling these questions using brain scans.

Science fiction or not?

"I know how to find secrets from your mind, I know all the tricks!" So says Dominic Cobb, the main character in *Inception*, the movie that inspired Crystal Goh to take up the study of neuroscience. But can an MRI scan really "read" your brain? Can it reveal your strengths and weaknesses?

Certainly not to the extent portrayed in *Inception*. MRI scans cannot extract your deepest secrets from your brain, but they *can* identify which parts of your brain need work. What's more, you can actually make changes in your brain. Goh's Neuroprofile service aims to help you improve parts of the brain that, for example, manage emotion regulation, or your high-level cognitive abilities.

So perhaps this doesn't sound like science fiction after all. A brain scan may well be worth considering as one method to help you become more self-aware and identify areas for improvement. That's if Crystal Goh can overcome the initial challenges in setting up her business. She will need to find a way around the regulatory hurdles discussed in this chapter. But perhaps the biggest challenge for Goh will be to convince consumers—you and me—that brain scans aren't scary and they do have value. While brain scans are common in Japan, they are far from common in the US and other parts of the Western world. Everywhere except Japan, brain scans are more likely to be feared than desired.

Neuroprofile will need to overcome the natural reticence that people have about MRI scans and (more particularly) the "brain stimulation" that may form part of the treatment. For Neuroprofile to work, somehow Crystal Goh will need to implant the idea in people's heads that brain scanning is OK. Inception, anyone?

CHAPTER SEVEN

BACTERIA NATION: TRACKING THE MICROBIOME WITH UBIOME

I feel like so much more science—not just the microbiome, but so many other things—can be used to measure what's actually going on.

Jessica Richman, co-founder and CEO of uBiome

I first met uBiome co-founder and CEO Jessica Richman at the grandly titled "Personalized Medicine World Conference," held late January 2013 in Mountain View, Silicon Valley. I'd been trying to track her down at the event, but she wasn't replying to my emails or text messages. Then I literally stumbled upon her in one of the busy hallways at the conference. A woman in her mid-twenties with a voluminous mass of curly blonde hair, she was kneeling on the floor and tapping nervously into a laptop computer. She looked flustered. Clearing my throat, I introduced myself and she looked up. "Oh, it's great to meet you," she said distractedly, her eyes returning immediately to the laptop, "but I have to do a presentation in ten minutes!" I wished her luck and we arranged to meet later that day.

Richman was about to present her young startup, uBiome, in a competition for "Most Promising Company" at the conference. uBiome is a similar service to the one offered by 23andMe, which I discussed in the previous chapter. Only instead of profiling *your* DNA, as 23andMe does, uBiome profiles the collective DNA of billions of micro-organisms inside your body—aka your microbiome. We're talking about microscopic organisms, such as the bacteria that live in your digestive system. Scientists estimate that the human body contains over ten times more microbial cells than human cells, so the microbiome is believed to be a critical part of overall health. The microbiome is particularly important for the health of our immune system and metabolism. But its influence could be much more—at least one study has posited that the microbiome helps regulate the nervous system.

Jessica Richman was nervous for a reason. uBiome was not only one of the newest startups at the Personalized Medicine World Conference, it hadn't even released its product yet. uBiome had only been announced to the public a couple of months before, in November 2012, when it launched a campaign to raise money on the crowdfunding platform Indiegogo. On the day we met, uBiome had so far raised $200,000 for its promising—yet so far nonexistent—service. Thousands of people had expressed interest, by pre-ordering a uBiome kit (including yours truly).

The scientific community is at the early stages of studying the microbiome and figuring out its significance in human health. All scientists know for sure is that you can't live without these micro-organisms. But they rely on you, as their host, just as much. In other words, the microbes in your body exist in a synergistic relationship with your body cells. The microbiome is complementary to your genome. Just as there was a project to map the human genome, there was a similar—if substantially smaller—effort to map the microbiome. The Human Microbiome Project (HMP) was launched in 2008 by the National Institutes of Health (NIH). The stated goal was to discover how changes in the human microbiome are associated with human health or disease. Although the project wrapped up in 2012, it's likely to be many years before the microbiome is fully understood—if it ever is.

One aspect of the microbiome couldn't be more different from the genome: our microbe tenants change, whereas our genes stay the same. So doing a microbiome test could become something we track over time, in much the same way that we might track our daily activity on a Fitbit. Indeed, this is a key part of uBiome's business plan.

Jessica Richman, tycoon in residence

I finally caught up with Jessica Richman after lunch at the conference. I spotted her mass of curly blonde hair inside one of the meeting rooms that adjoined the lunch area. She was still peering into her laptop, but I could see that she was browsing Twitter this time—checking for feedback about her presentation. As I entered the meeting room, she looked up and flashed a broad, welcoming smile. Her face was flushed and pink-cheeked, partly due to relief that the presentation was over, but also, I suspected, with the excitement of running a cutting-edge health technology company. Indeed, after just a few minutes of chatting, it was clear that Jessica Richman is one of those Silicon Valley residents who was destined to run a startup. What gave her away was her earnest personality, starting every sentence with "So ...," and having the gift of talking up a product that doesn't yet exist. In the weeks leading up to this conference, I'd seen a number of upbeat media profiles of uBiome. She had a knack of explaining what the microbiome was in ways that ordinary people would understand ("So, we are covered in bacterial cells and these bacteria are indicators of many things about our health"). Perhaps because of her youth and Silicon Valley talkativeness, Richman had already attracted controversy among the medical establishment by the time I interviewed her—something we'll get to later in this chapter.

Despite her relative youth, I discovered that Richman has an educational and work background that makes most of us look like high-school dropouts. After high school, she started and then quickly sold a startup (she wouldn't tell me the name of it, saying only that "it was a retail/wholesale operation"). Next she went to Stanford University, where she got a double degree in economics and computer science. After that, Oxford University in England, where she graduated with a master's in science specializing in network science and social entrepreneurship. She then began her PhD at Oxford, studying how new markets are formed. "It's mathematical sociology," she said by way of explanation. She paused, remembering that I come from the tech blogging world and not academia. "So, it's sort of like ... social network analysis." She has also attended the Graduate Summer Program at Singularity U—a Silicon Valley learning institution for extreme brainiacs, co-founded by NASA, Google, and other science and technology organizations. In the midst of all that study, Richman managed to get jobs at a couple of Silicon Valley venture capital firms, *and* at Google!

For uBiome Richman has partnered with two young scientists from the University of California, Dr. Will Ludington and Dr. Zachary Apte. "Will's a microbiologist and Zac is a biophysicist," said Richman. "They met doing microbiome research at UCSF." Richman met Apte first, at a startup event in Chile. He introduced her to Ludington and the three of them began talking about opportunities to commercialize the microbiome. "We launched our crowdfunding campaign in November 2012," she said, adding that they'd only started working on uBiome a month prior to that.

Richman explained that the genesis of the idea for uBiome came from the two microbiome scientists, Apte and Ludington. "So, they saw this microbiome research that they were doing and they thought, wouldn't it be awesome, let's sequence our microbiomes. But the problem is that, costwise, doing one microbiome was about the same as doing a hundred of them. So why not bring this technology to everyone." By "everyone," Richman means to make microbiome tests as common as DNA tests—which, if 23andMe's struggles are anything to go by, may not become mainstream for many years. But Richman is nothing if not a believer. Along with the Silicon Valley entrepreneur's gift for talking up her startup, Richman also has the supreme confidence of an over-qualified business school graduate.

How actionable is uBiome data?

In late November 2012, soon after uBiome launched its Indiegogo crowdfunding campaign, I contributed $79 to be a part of it. There were various levels of contributions and the one I signed up for was cutely labeled "uBiome Investigator." For my $79 contribution, I would get a microbiome kit for my GI tract and a T-shirt. As of August 2013, I still haven't received either. But when you sign up for an Indiegogo campaign, you expect delays and sometimes you may even forfeit your money.

Presuming I do eventually get a uBiome kit, how do I use it and what will it tell me? Whereas the 23andMe kit asked me to spit into a test tube, the uBiome kit will ask me to—there's no delicate way to put this—swab my bottom. The GI tract is your gut and so the sample you send back is of your excrement. The GI tract is the main microbiome testing area, as the gut is where the majority of micro-organisms in your body reside. But uBiome also offers microbiome tests for four other areas: your mouth, ears, nose, and genitalia. As with 23andMe, uBiome invites you to fill out an online survey to help it make correlations over time between test results and traits that people claim to have. Also like 23andMe, uBiome doesn't do a full sequence of your microbiome. uBiome does what is called "16S sequencing." Basically this is a sampling of a particular type of gene, called a "ribosomal gene," that is common in bacterial DNA. Analyzed this way, the bacteria in your body can be classified and compared.

According to the uBiome website, the results of your microbiome test will tell you "what lives in your gut (or other sampling area) at the time the sample was taken, and in what proportions." This so-called "microbiome profile" tells you what kinds of bacteria live in you and how this compares to other people—either other uBiome customers or those sourced from published scientific reports. The promotional video for uBiome on Indiegogo informs us that in the gut, which as noted is where many bacteria live, there are "usually around 200 prevalent species [of microbes] and up to 1,000 less common ones."

uBiome gives you visual tools to help explain your microbiome profile. In the gut test, you're assigned one of three "enterotypes," which is a classification of bacteria ecosystems in the gut microbiome. The enterotype classifications were announced as recently as April 2011 in *Nature* magazine. It's similar in a way to how blood was classified into four distinct types—A, B, AB, and O—in the early 1900s. The April 2011 announcement was that there are three distinct ecosystems of bacteria in the gut. "Blood type, meet bug type," as the *New York Times* put it. So what does your enterotype tell you? That's still relatively unknown; however, early studies have shown a correlation with diet. uBiome will tell you that if your enterotype is "Prevotella," for example, then that is "associated strongly with a long-term carbohydrate-heavy diet."

Your uBiome results will also show you a "Diversity Index," which compares your microbiome profile with those of other people and puts you into one of the following groups: "Healthy People;" "Mild Gut Disease;" "Severe Gut Disease." Basically, the more diverse the types of microbes in your gut, the more chance you have of some form of gut disease.

We saw in Chapter Five how 23andMe results can be contentious and not very actionable. This is even more so with uBiome results. A big reason is that the microbiome is a newer field of study than the human genome. Also bear in mind that although the human genome was mapped at the start of this century, it's still to this day poorly understood. So that uncertainty is multiplied when it comes to the microbiome.

In a nutshell, very little of your uBiome results will be actionable data at this time. Perhaps if you have made a significant change to your diet recently you can track it over time by testing your microbiome every few years. Jessica Richman acknowledged to me that it's still early days. However, she argues that the test could be useful to you in at least a few other ways. "One is that if you correlate very highly with someone who has a medical condition that you don't think you have," she told me earnestly, "maybe you should look into it. If you correlate 98.3% with type 2 diabetics and you have some symptoms, but you haven't been to a doctor, then I think you should go to the doctor."

Richman also mentioned the current trend among fitness fanatics to drink probiotic cocktails with live bacteria in them, which theoretically makes you healthier. "It won't be too far off before you'll be able to say, 'I need more of this bacteria and less of that,'" Richman said. In other words, you'll be able to "refresh your microbiome," as she put it. "I think having a test done now," she concluded, "will establish a baseline for these sorts of things."

Richman may be onto something with the probiotic example. The probiotics market has steadily increased over time, although it's mostly because of probiotic dairy products, like yogurt, rather than fitness drinks. According to a report published at the end of July 2013 by market research company MarketsandMarkets, the probiotic market was valued at $24.23 billion in 2011. Probiotic dairy products accounted for almost 80% of that total. The report stated that the probiotic market will grow by 6.8% every year from 2012 to 2017. "Rising levels of health consciousness" is given as one of the primary reasons for the growth of probiotics.

Probiotics make you healthier because they help the regulation of your gut, mouth, and other areas where bacteria thrive. Microbiome scientists are confident they will be able to identify many more types of bacteria that have health benefits than are currently known today.

In a June 2013 article in the web resource Medscape, Dr. Scott Peterson, Professor at the Infectious and Inflammatory Disease Center at Sanford-Burnham Medical Research Institute, pointed to the sheer number of genes in the microbiome as one source of optimism for this. "When we consider that the human genome has something of the order of 30,000 genes encoded," said Dr. Peterson, "the typical microbiome in a particular body site, such as the oral cavity or the human gut, will encode three million to ten million genes." So Dr. Peterson and his colleagues who are working on microbiome research believe that their chances are high of discovering links not

One future scenario is using the microbiome as a health supplement.

only to disease, but also "the potential for harvesting the health benefits of the microbiome."

One future scenario is using the microbiome as a health supplement, much as many of us take vitamins today to give us a health edge. Dr. Peterson continued, "We need to develop methods and mechanisms for identifying which microbes are producing therapeutic compounds—those that can improve human health or help to maintain human health, in the same way that we think of vitamins and herbal remedies helping to sustain human health."

The skeptics

uBiome has hitched its wagon firmly to the "citizen science" cause, which is a challenge to the traditional way of doing science. Citizen science typically uses public participation as the main driver of its research. Often it will be funded by so-called crowdfunding platforms like Indiegogo and Kickstarter. uBiome certainly qualifies in that respect, as it was launched on Indiegogo and raised $350,000 within a matter of months.

Some citizen science efforts are run by amateur or nonprofessional scientists, which tends to attract a lot of criticism from those in the scientific establishment. However, two of uBiome's three founders have science PhDs, so it has solid science credentials. That hasn't stopped it from being assailed by criticism though, from both the scientific establishment and science bloggers. Much of the attack has focused squarely on its nonscientist founder, Jessica Richman. Part of the problem has been Richman's hyperbolic promotion of uBiome. This is very common among Silicon Valley CEOs, who always claim to be "super excited" by whatever product or service their startup promotes. Richman, who proudly describes herself on the uBiome website as a "serial entrepreneur," clearly models herself more on Steve Jobs than Stephen Hawking. That's led to friction with the science establishment, which relies on rigorous evidential guidelines and a formal system of academic citations.

One of Richman's sharpest critics is Dr. Judy Stone, an

infectious disease specialist from Maryland and author of a book entitled *Conducting Clinical Research*. Dr. Stone writes a blog column for the magazine *Scientific American* and in a July 2013 article she took aim at uBiome. Her article began provocatively: "uBiome's CEO, Jessica Richman, seems to me to be a great saleswoman who also excels at sounding innocent and playing the misunderstood victim in the ethical controversy surrounding her company." The "ethical controversy" that Dr. Stone refers to is the lack of a formal review system in uBiome. In Dr. Stone's view, the claims that Jessica Richman makes for uBiome are "untested" and reflect "a desire for expediency over more careful volunteer protections." In other words, Dr. Stone thinks uBiome isn't proper science.

To summarize her concerns, Dr. Stone quotes another science blogger, Dr. Melissa Bates, who is a scientist in pediatric critical care medicine at the University of Wisconsin School of Medicine and Public Health. In her own very pointed blog post, Dr. Bates listed seven specific concerns about uBiome:

1. Participation in the uBiome project requires the payment of a fee.
2. There is no clear statement about what will be done with the data or samples.
3. There is no apparent plan for how your identity will be protected.
4. It's not clear what conflicts [of interest] the major players in the project might have.
5. The benefits you'll receive are grossly overstated.
6. There is no statement as to what your risks of participation are.
7. Children are included, but it's not apparent how they are protected.

In response to these concerns, Jessica Richman told me that points 2, 3, 6, and 7 are all false. "The information that refutes those points can be found on our website for anyone to read," she said.

Of particular interest to this book, which is about self-tracking, is the fifth of Dr. Bates' points. Are the claims by Jessica Richman grossly overstated? This is similar to criticism that has been aimed at 23andMe ever since it launched in 2007, culminating in the FDA sending 23andMe a warning letter in November 2013 about its marketing tactics. When I interviewed Jessica Richman in January 2013 for this book, she struggled to name clear, actionable benefits to doing a microbiome test. Being able to better determine the makeup of your probiotic cocktail seemed to be the biggest benefit she could name. But I would stop short of saying this is grossly overstating the benefits of uBiome. If Jessica Richman is guilty of anything, it's being overly optimistic—in that typical Silicon Valley CEO way—about how fast the science around the microbiome will progress.

Dr. Bates also took issue with this statement on uBiome's website: "uBiome is not a diagnostic test. However, we can give you valuable information about your microbiome that you can use to learn more about your health. You and your doctor can discuss the results of the test and determine the best way to proceed." Dr. Bates is skeptical that doctors will be able to make use of microbiome data at this time. She consulted a few of her physician colleagues and "they agree that they are not sure how they would use this data, if at all." This criticism I absolutely agree with. Again, it's a similar situation to 23andMe, which also is not a diagnostic test. Both services, uBiome and 23andMe, are offered direct to consumers. They aren't tests prescribed by or done through your doctor or a hospital. A big reason for that is that the scientific community still knows relatively little about how to interpret genetic and microbiome data.

As for the other ethical concerns outlined by Drs. Stone and Bates, uBiome will need to address those in time—if it hasn't already done so—for the protection of its customers. It's a young startup, led by a highly educated but still pretty green CEO. To be taken seriously by consumers and the medical establishment alike, uBiome needs to adhere to the ethical codes of the science establishment.

What are the benefits of crowdsourcing?

All the health technology startups profiled in this book rely on crowdsourcing to varying degrees. For example, the Fitbit dashboard lets you compare your activity level to those of people in your age group, which is anonymous data sourced from all of Fitbit's users. MyFitnessPal's huge database of food information is predominantly sourced from its 40 million users. uBiome will also gather data from its community in this manner.

The flip side of crowdsourcing for health technology companies is that it grates with the medical establishment. That's because traditionally, health information has been controlled by doctors and hospitals. To this day, most of us do not have electronic access to our own medical records (a subject I'll explore in depth in upcoming chapters). But the paternalism of the medical establishment is slowly changing, thanks in no small measure to direct-to-consumer services like uBiome and 23andMe. These are services that not only provide their customers with very personal health data, but also gather information from them (aka crowdsourcing). The first consumer health company to seriously challenge the medical research establishment in this way was 23andMe. Since uBiome models itself closely on 23andMe, it's worth turning our attention again to 23andMe to examine its approach to crowdsourcing.

One of the biggest corporate goals of 23andMe is to find answers to the many questions about genetic data by aggregating as much user data as possible. This is why 23andMe reduced its pricing below $100 in December 2012. Its desire to reach one million customers is less about increasing revenue than about increasing data. The more customers 23andMe has, the more genetic data it has, the more correlations it can make between data, and the more answers it can provide to thorny genetic questions. In an open letter published in the Quantified Self blog in December 2012, 23andMe CEO Anne Wojcicki noted that 23andMe's customers have "helped us create a novel research platform." In other words, it's research driven by crowdsourcing of data. Wojcicki isn't just referring to the results of genetics tests, but also to the surveys 23andMe users regularly fill out on the website. At the October 2012 Health 2.0 Conference in San Francisco, Wojcicki claimed that its users contribute one million new survey answers every week.

Wojcicki has been known to brag about how much more effective 23andMe's crowdsourcing approach to research is than the traditional citation-based approach. Her biggest cheerleader is none other than her husband, Google co-founder Sergey Brin (although the couple separated in 2013). Not only was Google an early investor in 23andMe, but Brin himself has been an alpha user and investor.

In September 2008, Sergey Brin started a blog in which he discussed his genetic predisposition to Parkinson's disease. He wrote that through 23andMe he discovered that he had a gene mutation that was highly correlated with Parkinson's. The gene in question is known as LRRK2 and the mutation has been labeled G2019S. Brin also found via 23andMe that his mother, who had previously developed the symptoms of Parkinson's, also had the mutation. What really intrigued Brin is the possibility of rapidly advancing the research into Parkinson's using 23andMe data. He contributed $4 million of his own money to help fund an online Parkinson's Disease Genetics Initiative at 23andMe. Launched in March 2009, the initiative aimed to sign up 10,000 people who had been diagnosed with Parkinson's disease. These people would contribute their genetic data, as well as fill out surveys about their family history, disease progression, treatment response, and environmental exposures. According to 23andMe at the time, "this effort will serve as a model for supporting research in many other diseases."

So how is this different from the traditional way of doing research? For one, conventional research projects typically involve far fewer volunteers than 10,000. If they get 2,000 volunteers, that's a huge effort. And the time it takes to analyze the data and present it is much quicker with 23andMe's model. It's also less robust, of course—and this is the main objection of Jessica Richman's chief critic, Dr. Judy Stone. This gets to the nub of the issue. The key concern with crowdsourced science is that much of the data is self-reported by individuals, without the rigid reporting structure of a conventional research project. Instead of being monitored by a group of white-coated scientists, the 10,000 participants in 23andMe's Parkinson's initiative simply fill out online surveys. Who knows how many of 23andMe's 10,000 customers are reliable?

Like Wojcicki, Jessica Richman also makes bold claims about how effective uBiome's crowdsourcing approach is compared to conventional studies into the microbiome. Richman gleefully told me that the NIH project, The Human Microbiome Project, only had 250 participants. "I mean it's just ridiculous how small that was," she chuckled. She checked herself, wiped the smile off her face and turned serious again. "It's an amazing project and it was groundbreaking what they were doing," she continued earnestly, "but by going directly to the public, you can do so much more." At time of writing, uBiome has 2,500 people signed up to take a microbiome test. That's ten times the number of people who did the NIH test.

Predictably, scientists have taken issue with Richman's pooh-poohing of the NIH project. They rightly point out that the NIH project was much more rigorously conducted than what uBiome is proposing. Also, only 250 participants were needed at the time in the NIH project for the purposes of furthering microbiome science. Fair enough, but what did the scientific community learn from the five-year US$173-million Human Microbiome Project, completed in mid-2012? As with the human genome study that was completed at the turn of the century, the microbiome project successfully sequenced the microbes that live on and inside our bodies. A *Nature* magazine wrap-up of the project in June 2012 reported that from a study of 242 US adults, researchers had "determined the whole-genome sequences of about 800 bacterial strains isolated from humans (from a planned total of 3,000)." Despite falling short of the 3,000 bacteria expected to be sequenced when the project began, the team concluded that it had "identified the majority of the common microbial taxa and their genes present in these 242 healthy humans."

Much as the human genome was successfully mapped after the turn of this century, so the Human Microbiome Project was successful in gathering and classifying a lot of new data about microbial genomes. However, also like the human genome project, the microbiome project failed to uncover much in the way of actionable knowledge. "Studying the human microbiome has so far been a lesson in humility," concluded the *Nature* article. Although the project "revealed vast amounts of previously uncharacterized microbial diversity within our 'home turf' [i.e. the human body], the functions of these communities remain largely unknown."

> Like the human genome project, the microbiome project failed to uncover much in the way of actionable knowledge.

At the end of July 2013, *Nature* magazine reiterated that "identifying the microbes is just the first step." It noted that "researchers must also focus on how bacteria interact with each other and the human body to cause—or prevent—disease." Lita Proctor, the program director of the Human Microbiome Project, is, rather ominously, quoted as saying that scientists are still "struggling to figure out how to think about the microbiome." Another point worth noting is that even if scientists did find more links between the microbiome and human disease, they probably wouldn't know what to do with that knowledge. As Professor Jonathan Eisen from the University of California, Davis, told NPR: "We don't know how to fix a microbiome, even if we knew what was wrong with it."

uBiome may well contribute to the scientific landscape of microbiome research, at least in terms of adding more data. However, it is unlikely to speed up the long process of finding answers to the hundreds of questions that NIH-funded scientists are grappling with. Where the uBiome project still holds potential value for self-trackers lies in the fact that at least you can try it out for yourself. Rather than rely on the official scientific studies, which are far from complete, you can do a uBiome test and discover what microbes are residing in your body—as long as you're willing to take on the privacy risks that Dr. Judy Stone and others have rightly identified about uBiome. Also, don't expect many insights at this point in time. It will take the conventional scientists *and* citizen scientists alike a number of years more to come to their conclusions.

The edge of possible

Even Jessica Richman, for all of her hyperbolic startup talk and breezy dismissals of the NIH, admits that the microbiome world is "on the edge of possible" at this time. "I think the future is kind of crazy," she told me in January of 2013 at the Personalized Medicine conference in Silicon Valley. "The future is sensors in your toilet that know exactly what's going on with you," she said—a polite way of saying that your future toilet will analyze your poo.

"The future is targeted probiotics that make you skinny," Richman continued. "Crazy ideas that are on the edge of possible. Either slightly impossible, or possible, but not yet at scale. So I think there's a lot of really interesting stuff that will happen. Like one thing we've been thinking about a lot is that your tool for measuring weight loss is, what, a scale? Some calipers, maybe? That's it, right? I feel like so much more science—not just the microbiome, but so many other things—can be used to measure what's actually going on."

As we've discovered so far in this book, there is a dichotomy between what you can track and finding practical uses for it. The microbiome is the starkest reminder yet of that, although as we've seen there is also a big gap between the amount of genetic data you can discover about yourself and the usefulness of that data. However, one way all of these different types of self-tracking we've discussed so far—activity, food, weight, genetics, microbiome—might yield more usable insights is to merge them together.

In the next chapter I'll profile a dashboard product called TicTrac, which aims to do precisely this. But I was curious to hear Jessica Richman's view on that. Will uBiome customers be able to mix their microbiome data with their Fitbit data, their 23andMe data, and so on?

"Yeah, we hope to," she replied. "I mean, not in our first version, but we want to be able to integrate with 23andMe, integrate with Fitbit and diet apps, tracking apps and all these sorts of things—because it just makes sense." She sees uBiome data as just "another source of data" for tracking your daily health over time. She's also keen to integrate uBiome data with medical data. "On the medical side, we want to be able to integrate with blood tests and with parasitology tests and all sorts of other things." She thinks this will enable physicians and health professionals to test for a certain condition "from different angles."

Another avenue that uBiome will explore is utilizing social media. Jessica Richman thinks this is another area where the citizen science approach has benefits. "We want people to be able to ask and answer questions of the data," she told me. She envisions groups of people forming on social networks like Facebook and Twitter to undertake specific experiments. For example, continued Richman, someone might start a public group on Facebook looking for 50 volunteers to do the uBiome gut test, in order to see what effect various probiotics have on their bodies. The group might do the uBiome test before the experiment starts, then again during the experiment, and finally after it's finished. "Let's all test it!" said Richman enthusiastically, "and we'll see what happens." For Jessica Richman, citizen science is all about the data. The Facebook experiment described above will at the very least contribute more microbiome data to the world. "If thousands of people run their own little experiments, we all benefit from that knowledge." The keyword, other than data, is collaboration. "Let's all collaborate to be scientists together," Richman said, with her best Silicon Valley CEO optimistic smile.

So what's the role of your doctor in all of this? Jessica Richman thinks your family doctor will have to adapt from being a provider of information to someone who helps you analyze it. "Right now, you go to the doctor and they tell you things you don't know. Whereas I think as the shift [to self-tracking] occurs, you go to the doctor with all your information and they'll help you make sense of it." She compared this new type of doctor to a financial planner, who helps you interpret and make sense of all of your financial data. "You're going to be giving them information," said Richman, "and then they'll use their expertise and their training to tell you what to make of it."

Of course, that scenario will depend on the scientific community coming up with more answers and actionable information about the microbiome. Asking your doctor to be your microbiome advisor at the present time would be like expecting your financial planner to give you advice about foreign exchange derivatives in the currency market. It's unlikely she will know about those types of derivatives; and even if she does, it'll be highly speculative advice.

Overcoming the obstacles

The state of microbiome science in many ways mirrors the background and personality of Jessica Richman, the vivacious and super-smart Silicon Valley entrepreneur, Oxford University graduate, and alumna of Google. Both are very young and relatively untested in the real world—by which I mean the world outside of Silicon Valley and Ivy League universities. Yet Richman is undoubtedly full of promise, much like the microbiome. For this reason I find it hard not to share in her enthusiasm for her microbiome startup, even if much of what she says is speculative or even—if you're a hard-boiled, old-fashioned scientist—objectionable.

But let's take a step back. Throughout the writing of this book, I've tried to imagine if my mostly non-techie relatives would use the tools I'm talking about. The signs aren't good at this point in time. As I noted in Chapter Five, just one of my three siblings has so far done a 23andMe test—even though I offered to pay for it. I also don't think any of my family would rush out to use a Fitbit or the smartphone app MyFitnessPal. Of all the startup products profiled in this book, uBiome would be the least likely to be used by my family.

There are two main obstacles that self-tracking products face at the present time. The first obstacle is that the data these products provide has limited applicability currently. uBiome is an extreme example of this. Right now, what you would learn from a microbiome test is not something you can use to make an improvement in your lifestyle. You can't even take it to your doctor, because it's highly unlikely she will know how to interpret it. That said, some of the other products I've written up in this book can be used to make meaningful changes in your lifestyle right now. For example, your Fitbit can motivate you to keep active every day and MyFitnessPal helps you stick to a diet. But even those examples have relatively limited usefulness, especially when you consider the second obstacle for self-tracking products.

This second obstacle is that the current generation of products don't fit seamlessly into our daily lives and aren't part of our regular health checkups. Certainly that's the case with microbiome tests, which aren't something a doctor would prescribe or that many of us would think to purchase. But let's use the Fitbit as an example, as that's more mainstream at the time I write this. The Fitbit is a sophisticated and highly capable little device. You slip it in the pocket of your jeans, or clip it on your bra. Yet even the Fitbit isn't a particularly seamless fit for our everyday lives. You have to remember to put it on every morning; in my own experience, I've often forgotten to do so. You have to be careful not to leave your Fitbit on your clothing at night as it may end up in your washing machine (my first one lasted just a week or two before suffering that fate). You have to sync your Fitbit and charge it every now and then. If you change your clothes during the day, sometimes you'll forget to put your Fitbit on again, which messes up your daily step count.

So if self-tracking products—and uBiome is the most extreme example of this right now—don't provide enough actionable data and don't fit seamlessly into our lives at the present time ... then why am I writing this book? Because the data will become more useful, the products will become more seamless. It's a matter of time. The fact that we can get this data *at all* right now—everything from accurate daily steps data, to information about our food intake, to a profile of our DNA, to a scan of our microbiome—is a huge step in itself in medical science. It's what excites entrepreneurs like Jessica Richman, that they are able to offer ordinary people (you and me) a chance to gather a new kind of data about our own bodies.

The next step, of course, is to make sense of that data, to make it useful in monitoring our daily health, whether to prevent disease (the primary focus of 23andMe) or to implement meaningful change in our lifestyles (the focus of Fitbit and MyFitnessPal). All the other products I've written about so far in this book—23andMe, Fitbit, and MyFitnessPal— are further down that data interpretation track than uBiome. But even they have a long way to go. As for uBiome, its main challenge is that scientists are still in the very early days of making sense of microbiome data, earlier even than is the case with human genomics.

Preventing disease and making lifestyle changes are what we need these self-tracking products to help us with. Jessica Richman has to believe that those connections will come. It's the brass ring she's reaching for as a Silicon Valley entrepreneur. If she grabs it, we'll all be the better off for it.

CHAPTER EIGHT

THE HEALTH DASHBOARD: TICTRAC

Our mission is to empower people through their own data.

Martin Blinder, co-founder and CEO of TicTrac

When 37-year-old Londoner Martin Blinder visited his doctor at the beginning of 2013, he asked him to open up his Web browser and go to the Web address tictrac.com.

"May I?" asked Blinder, nodding at the doctor's computer keyboard to indicate that he'd like to log in. "Of course," smiled his doctor, leaning back in his chair. Blinder stood up, leaned in front of the doctor, and tapped his username and password into the computer. As he sat back down, Martin Blinder's health dashboard appeared on his doctor's screen. The TicTrac website was a vibrant mix of bright blues, punchy purples, resilient reds, and calming charcoals. It made a stark contrast to the doctor's own medical records for Blinder, which the pair had been viewing just minutes before. The doctor's default screen was a mass of sickly green type on a dull black background. Blinder had winced when he saw it—it was like looking at a computer from the 80s! But he couldn't help but smile now as the beautifully designed TicTrac website glowed in front of them. He thought he spotted the doctor's eyes widening slightly in appreciation.

The doctor moved his mouse around the colorful TicTrac display, surveying data that included Blinder's weight, blood pressure readings, stress levels, calories consumed, his runs, and even the daily weather. Blinder watched his transfixed doctor for a minute before showing him how to compare two sets of data and graph it. Following Blinder's careful instructions, the doctor graphed his patient's blood pressure and how it correlated with daily stress. "Where did those readings come from?" the doctor asked, looking somewhat mystified. Blinder explained that the blood pressure readings came from a device by a startup called Withings. "It's called a Withings Blood Pressure Monitor," he continued, "and it's basically the same as the inflatable arm band you use. Only it has a connector to my iPhone, so I can export the readings." He pointed to the website. "They show up in TicTrac too, because my phone sends the data to the Cloud … er, I mean the Internet." The doctor nodded and turned back to the computer monitor. He pointed at the stress data. "How do you get that data then?" Pulling out his iPhone, Blinder showed the doctor how he manually inputs a stress reading every day into the TicTrac iPhone app. "Unlike the blood pressure," he said, a little apologetically, "the stress data is subjective." He tapped the iPhone screen and looked earnestly at his GP. "Every day I measure my stress level on a scale of one to five." The doctor smiled at Blinder and tipped his head toward the computer. "Seems like running a startup is a stressful business, eh?"

The dashing Martin Blinder

It was a cold, drizzly winter evening in January when Martin Blinder and I met for dinner at the upmarket BobBobRicard restaurant in Soho, London. Blinder was tall, with close-cropped, thick dark hair and designer stubble. He was stylishly dressed in a dark blue sweater and black dress trousers. As we shook hands, it occurred to me that he wouldn't look out of place on a *GQ* cover.

Martin Blinder is the co-founder and CEO of London-based startup TicTrac. His company's product is a dashboard for people to track various things about their lives, from their health to their computer habits to their daily spending. The blood pressure and stress readings that Blinder had shown his doctor are just a couple of the many data types TicTrac can monitor. At the time of our interview, in January 2013, TicTrac was connected to 45 different services—such as the Internet scale Withings, activity tracker Fitbit, and food logging app FatSecret. There are eight different running apps alone. But there are dozens more running apps available, and I got the impression that Martin Blinder wants TicTrac to connect to them all.

Blinder is in many ways an ideal startup CEO. He's photogenic, like Twitter co-founder Jack Dorsey. He's also very talkative, like Dallas Mavericks owner (and former dot com entrepreneur) Mark Cuban. I marveled that Blinder talked in full sentences, without ums and ahs. There was only one slightly strange thing about him: he has an indeterminate accent. It's not British, not American … The accent was the one thing about him I couldn't place. It wasn't till the main course that I finally asked him where the accent comes from. Laughing, he replied that he hasn't figured it out yet either. He explained that he's Argentinian, but he was brought up in the US and then spent eight years in Spain in his twenties.

Blinder's parents immigrated to the US in 1980, when he was five, because of the military dictatorship in Argentina. His father is IT Director at the United Nations, so the boy attended United Nations schools in New York City. "I mixed with a lot of international kids," he remarked, perhaps explaining his hard-to-pin-down accent. Along with a geographically diverse background, Martin Blinder has been steeped in the medical world from an early age. "Most of my family are doctors," he said, noting that his sister is an oncologist in New York City. His parents aren't medical doctors, although his mother is a speech pathologist and his paternal grandfather was an MD. Many of his extended family are in the medical profession. "My uncles and aunts and half my cousins are MDs," he told me, "so medicine has always been woven into conversations at family gatherings."

Martin Blinder himself went on to major in economics at Trinity College in Hartford, Connecticut. "I'm the only commercial one," he chuckled. After graduating, Blinder took the route of many financial graduates in America: he became a management consultant. But after just a year and a half in that role, in the middle of the dot com boom, the startup bug bit. He co-founded a financial services website in Spain called Tuhipoteca.com. "My very first taste of data," is how Blinder describes his dot com experience. Tuhipoteca taught Blinder about using data to "generate a better understanding of consumer behavior." However, the world of finance was a "stilted environment," he said ruefully, similar perhaps to the bureaucratic and still largely paternalistic medical establishment today.

The evolution of TicTrac

A few years after Tuhipoteca, a former colleague started a "data-oriented digital agency" in the UK called Essence. Blinder joined Essence and it was here, in early 2008, that he and new workmate Oliver MacCarthy came up with the initial idea for TicTrac. They were working on a project for Google at that time.

Blinder and MacCarthy's job was to come up with ideas for Google's online dashboard product. Called iGoogle, it was one of Google's many experiments as it tried to expand into areas other than search. iGoogle was a webpage populated with interactive boxes called "gadgets." These gadgets, also known in the industry as "widgets," were basically mini Web applications. They each had a specific functionality, such as displaying the latest weather, showing your unread email, delivering news feeds, or being a calculator. Each gadget connected to an external service, such as the Weather Channel, or an email client like Google's own Gmail.

Google hoped that iGoogle would become a personalized homepage for its users. It would be a site to visit each morning to take care of multiple tasks—check email, see the weather forecast, browse the latest headlines, and so on. For this reason, iGoogle and similar products came to be known as "start pages." Start pages were something all the big players on the Internet at that time were trying. Microsoft had one called Live.com and Yahoo had a popular webpage called MyYahoo. Perhaps the best of them was a trendy startup called Netvibes, which pioneered the concept in 2005. Bear in mind that all of this was playing out over 2005 to 2008, before Facebook became overwhelmingly popular. Back then, becoming the webpage where people began their day was a market very much up for grabs.

Unfortunately for Google and the other contenders, start pages ultimately failed to capture the public imagination. For a start, they were too geeky—people didn't want to set up "gadgets" or "widgets," or whatever strange name these odd little boxes were given by the likes of Google and Microsoft. Also, the start pages tended to run slowly and gadgets sometimes failed. Yahoo was perhaps the most successful at integrating gadgets into a popular product. Its MyYahoo! webpage was well used and integrated nicely with Yahoo's news and email products. But it also had less connectivity to external services than Netvibes, iGoogle, and Microsoft's Live.com. That was a big part of the appeal of dashboards, pulling in content from elsewhere on the Web. MyYahoo! was more of a traditional Internet portal. Most of its content was Yahoo-branded and designed to keep users in the Yahoo world.

Both Google and Microsoft eventually shuttered their start pages. The French startup Netvibes failed to gain consumer traction too, after its initial take-up by early adopters. Netvibes was eventually sold to an enterprise company and morphed into a social media analytics tool. Ultimately of course, Facebook usurped all of these products and became the start page of choice for a billion people worldwide.

Regardless of the eventual demise of the "start page" market, online dashboards did—and still do—have a future. Martin Blinder and Oliver MacCarthy recognized this after the Essence team created various gadgets for iGoogle in 2008. As Martin Blinder explained to *Wired UK* in February 2012, "One of the apps [developed for iGoogle] was an alcohol awareness tool which enabled users to keep track of their alcohol consumption and see how many calories they were consuming from drinking." The gadget enabled users to track how many calories they consumed from alcohol each day. "That's when the idea struck," said Blinder. "What if you could do this for any aspect of your life?"

Blinder and MacCarthy brought in a third co-founder, developer James Pollock, and together they began fleshing out the product that would eventually become TicTrac. TicTrac today is a browser-based dashboard of various bits of personal data—everything from health, to work, to social media, and more. Each data type can be made into what TicTrac calls a "tracker." For example, if you want to track your weight, you'll create a "My Weight" tracker (although you can name it anything you like). You can either manually input the data into the tracker, or connect the tracker to a third-party service. In the case of weight, there are currently five services to choose from: FatSecret, Fitbit (via the Aria scale discussed earlier), RunKeeper, Medisana, or Withings (the product Amelia Greenhall uses, covered in Chapter Four). If you choose to connect one of those five, your weight readings are automatically updated into TicTrac.

A collection of "trackers" is called a "project," which is the main organizing principle behind TicTrac. For example, your weight tracker can be combined with other health-related trackers to form a project called "My Health." Along with weight, you could also be tracking your blood pressure, your stress levels, how many steps you walk a day, what you eat, runs or swims taken, and more. This is what Martin Blinder showed his doctor in early 2013, a project that included health data such as blood pressure readings and stress ratings.

TicTrac enables you to track whatever you want, from whatever tool you want.

Blinder told me that people live their lives in projects. "Their careers, having kids, travel. All of these things (and much more) can be viewed as projects," he said. What TicTrac has done is build a self-tracking dashboard around that concept. It's a tool to project-manage your life, Blinder explained—or at least the parts of your life that might benefit from better management.

In summary then, TicTrac enables you to track whatever you want, from whatever tool you want. Things that you track are organized into projects and these are viewable in one place on the Web, the TicTrac dashboard.

The age of insights

I first became of aware of TicTrac at an annual health technology conference in San Francisco, Health 2.0. At this event, in October 2012, TicTrac debuted its product to a crowd of healthcare industry professionals and technology enthusiasts. At that time TicTrac was in a private beta, meaning that only a limited number of people had been given access. Martin Blinder showed off TicTrac in a short presentation as part of a startup competition called "Launch!" The contest was billed as "a series of rapid-fire, back-to-back, 3.5 minute demos from new, buzz-worthy companies making their debut at Health 2.0."

"We live life in little projects," began Blinder in his presentation. Because he was pressed for time, he focused on the visualization of personal data in TicTrac—including the ability to correlate two pieces of data in a graph. He used the same blood pressure and stress example that he'd previously shown his doctor. Although the presentation went smoothly, ironically it bumped up his stress level for that day. The time limit made it "the most stressful presentation you can do," Blinder told me a few months later. But it paid off. TicTrac won the Health 2.0 Launch! competition, which earned the London startup early media attention and prestige among its health technology peers.

I got in touch with Blinder soon after the Health 2.0 event and began to hound him for an invite to TicTrac, which hadn't yet opened to the public. Eventually I got to play with the product in January 2013, a few weeks before I met Blinder in person in London. I was impressed with the design and the ability to track data about myself. The product was clearly in its early days and there were some bugs—for example, my Fitbit data updated erratically. But that's to be expected in a private beta. I could see the potential in this.

Although TicTrac was inspired by the mini Web apps in the iGoogle dashboard, Martin Blinder is adamant that TicTrac will be more than just a dashboard. He argues that products like iGoogle and Netvibes failed because they gave users too much information, which overwhelmed them.

Martin Blinder wants to help people organize the information in their dashboard into manageable projects. He's even coined a phrase for this (I discovered, over dinner, that coining new marketing phrases is a hobby of Blinder's). "TicTrac," he announced, prodding his fork in my direction, "is a lifestyle design platform." Noting my confused look, Blinder tried to elaborate. "We don't live life in a silo, right? So what affects you in one aspect of your life will always affect you in another. You can't look at lowering your blood pressure in a vacuum. You've got to see what are the aspects of your life that could be causing the problem. Is it too much coffee? Could it be your baby crying a lot at nights, creating more stress? There are so many factors in life, so we wanted TicTrac to be a holistic type of platform."

This word "holistic" is often used by health startup CEOs and forward-looking healthcare practitioners, such as Dr. Robin Berzin (whom we will meet in the next chapter). It means that everything is interconnected, so the best system is one that looks at something by reference to the whole. What TicTrac is attempting is to be a platform where you have lots of different types of data flowing in (blood pressure readings, stress ratings, activity, weight, and so on). The idea is that you gain insights into your health by mixing all of that data together—by cross-referencing, for example, your blood pressure readings with your stress levels. In other words, TicTrac wants to not just be a way for people to track various pieces of data, but also to help you interpret that data.

Martin Blinder also wants to bring in experts to help. TicTrac hopes to entice specialists to use its platform and offer their services. In the healthcare market, that would be professionals like personal trainers, doctors, and nutritionists. Blinder calls this a "contextual layer" on top of a person's health and lifestyle data. Dipping back into his marketing playbook, Blinder told me that a "lifestyle marketplace" will develop. "We've created a marketplace, and that marketplace brings together those people [personal trainers, doctors, nutritionists, and other experts]. So as a user, I continuously generate more and more data. We believe that the market is going toward a world where at a certain point, I'm going to need context around that data. Otherwise it won't mean anything, right?"

In fact, Blinder goes as far as to say that the user may not even need a dashboard view of her data. "I foresee the dashboard in TicTrac [being] an optional view," he explained. "What I want TicTrac to be is 'the world according to you.' So, the contextual content will be the more important aspect. That and the contact you've got with your doctor, your personal trainer, your nutritionist—who are actively sending you instructions or insights off of your data."

Branded

This all begs the question of how TicTrac will make money. Will TicTrac charge you a fee to have an expert interpret your data? Will it charge the service providers? Or maybe you'll have to look at those horrible "Lose 15 pounds now!!!" adverts with the before and after photos of freakish people? Not according to Martin Blinder. Predictably, he has a cunning plan for monetizing too—and it ties into TicTrac's mission to provide people with insights into their personal data.

Before I explain that, it helps to have a little context about how consumer Web services usually make money. Most consumer Web services are free to use. Think Google search or Gmail, Yahoo Finance, Facebook, and Twitter. The reason why most things are free on the Web is that we have all become very used to it, thanks to the advertising business model. Online advertising is how all that free stuff has been funded. Companies such as Google and Yahoo! make the majority of their revenue from advertising. And up to about 2011, that was the way almost all new startups in the consumer Web market made money, if indeed they made any money at all. Many startups are given wads of cash by venture capitalists in the hope that they will get millions of users and eventually be acquired. Most don't get millions of users. The very few that do, typically "monetize" their massive user base by putting ads on the site. That's how Google and Facebook became such valuable businesses. In the case of Google, for years its search product didn't have adverts. But as soon as Google had built up a sizable audience, it introduced AdWords—contextual adverts in search results—and the rest is history.

The advertising model began to break down somewhat with the arrival of the mobile Web. From the time Apple opened its iPhone App Store in July 2008, it became increasingly more difficult to make money from adverts, because there's less room for ads inside a mobile device. Plus, users tend to click less often on mobile ads anyway. Because people are using mobile devices for Internet services more and more every year, from about 2010 onward many consumer Web services started looking for other ways to make money. Fortunately, the mobile Web opened up an excellent alternative business model: subscriptions. Successful startups in the mobile Web era—like Evernote, Spotify and Dropbox—make a large proportion of their revenue through premium subscriptions. By purchasing a subscription (typically monthly or annual), a consumer gets a better experience: better mobile access, advanced functionality, and no ads.

However, subscriptions won't work for every type of consumer business. While TicTrac could offer a premium service—for example, with advanced visualization features— it would first need to build a sizable user base. This almost certainly would require running at a loss, since it's likely that running adverts alone wouldn't be enough to keep the business afloat without significant funding. In summary then, TicTrac needs a better way to build a business than relying on advertising and/or subscriptions.

Which brings us back to Martin Blinder's bright idea. He wants to marry TicTrac's vision to offer its users insights with the ability of brands to help offer those insights, in other words, branded projects that help you interpret your personal data and/or give you contextual content based on your data. The idea is that the brands will pay TicTrac for the privilege of accessing your data. Nothing is more valuable to big brands than personal data about their target audience.

According to Martin Blinder, brands fit naturally within their service. "There'll be dozens of projects like this," enthused Blinder. He gave an example of Gatorade, the energy sports drink, offering a branded project for runners. "Gatorade could help you run your first 10 kilometers!" he said eagerly, as if I was a Gatorade executive he was pitching to. I nodded doubtfully. Blinder switched to the point of view of a typical user. "Perhaps that's my New Year's resolution. So I sign up and see it's Gatorade offering me that project, but they're offering me something of value and so I gladly give them my running data within that spectrum." That "something of value" would be content personalized on the basis of his running data, for example, a video program that adapts to each level of his performance.

> **Brands will pay TicTrac for the privilege of accessing your data.**

The privacy question

You might be reading this and thinking, hang on, do I really want to give big brands like Gatorade, or McDonald's, or Coca-Cola, access to my personal data?

While you may get some value out of it, you're still essentially handing over what was previously private information about yourself to a corporation. What if Gatorade accidentally divulges your personal data? What if it sells your data to a health insurance company? Or uses your personal details in its advertising? These may all be low risks, but they are risks nonetheless.

These kinds of privacy issues have been a concern on the social Web for a few years now. It's always helpful to bring Facebook into discussions about privacy, since it's the world's largest social network and has come under pressure many times over this issue. If you are one of the billion-plus people on the planet who use Facebook, you've likely already input personal data into the site. The simple reason you did that is because you want to connect to your friends. That's the value that Facebook, the corporation, provides you: enter your personal data into our website and you'll keep up to date with what your friends are doing. If you join the Gatorade project on TicTrac, you're essentially doing the same thing: entering personal data with the intention of getting back information of value to you: in this case, insights and advice about your running data.

The problem is that you have very little control over what corporations do with your data. Indeed, Facebook itself has a poor track record of respecting its users' privacy. The most controversial example was an advertising system Facebook called Beacon. Introduced in November 2007, Beacon enabled Facebook to track purchases you made on partner websites (which at the time of launch included eBay and Sony Pictures) and publish that information in your news feed. The result was sometimes embarrassing for users, for example, when a purchase from eBay that was never meant to be public was automatically published to that person's Facebook wall. Facebook's biggest flub was not giving its users a way to opt out of Beacon. After mounting pressure, including lawsuits, Facebook announced just a month later that it would allow people to opt out of Beacon.

However, that didn't stop the controversy, because many people thought Beacon should be opt-in—requiring a Facebook user to give their explicit permission to allow Beacon to use their data. Opt-in is essentially an added layer of protection for the consumer, because it means external parties cannot access your personal data unless you permit it. Third-party access is turned off by default. It only gets turned on if you opt in to the Beacon service. Opt-out, on the other hand, means that external parties can access your data straight away. In other words, Beacon is turned on by default. So if you don't want it, then you have to go into your Facebook settings and explicitly turn it off. The trouble with opt-out is that the majority of people rarely—if ever—tweak the settings of services like Facebook. Most people stick with the default settings, so they may not even know that their data is being accessed by third parties.

Although Facebook relented on letting users opt out of Beacon, it refused to bow to pressure to make Beacon opt-in. The controversy didn't abate until Beacon was eventually shut down in September 2009.

In November 2011, Facebook CEO Mark Zuckerberg himself characterized Beacon as a privacy "mistake." The lesson, as always with consumer products, is caveat emptor: let the buyer beware. In the case of the Gatorade example in TicTrac, you do have to opt in to that project. So it does have that added layer of privacy protection. If you are at all concerned about what Gatorade might do with your personal data, then the solution is simple: don't opt in.

Privacy issues are a constant area of concern for Internet products. This will only become exacerbated as more and more of your data flows through the Internet, into rapidly increasing numbers of companies, and through many types of devices. For example, already your Fitbit data can flow through to TicTrac and you can access it on TicTrac's website and its iPhone app. Fitbit is one of 45 different services that currently plug into TicTrac. In a year or two, that number may be 145 and TicTrac may have new apps on devices such as Android phones, iPads, maybe even Internet TV sets. In other words, not only is personal data multiplying on the Web at an exponential rate, it's also becoming much more wide-ranging. Your personal data is increasingly being accessed by a range of Web services and across many different Internet-connected devices. As Martin Blinder described it to me, in another one of his buzzword-laden marketing phrases, it's an "interwoven ecosystem of data."

APIs

The changes to data flows on the Internet are both a huge opportunity for TicTrac, and a huge challenge. There are lots of moving parts in TicTrac: the users (who are, of course, the most important part); brands; service providers, such as doctors and nutritionists; and third-party services like Fitbit.

Of all those players in the budding TicTrac ecosystem, the most troublesome are the third-party services. This is because that part needs to be automated, so that—for example—my Fitbit data flows straight through to TicTrac's website without any leakages (missing data) or delays. This is where TicTrac relies on a piece of technology known as an API: Application Programming Interface. I won't bore you with the technical detail, but suffice to say an API is how your Fitbit data gets from Fitbit's servers to TicTrac's servers. The world of APIs is further complicated by the fact that TicTrac has no control over what data is sent, or when it's sent. What's more, the user herself has little control over that. Essentially, it's the third party (in our example, Fitbit) that controls what data it gives to TicTrac and when.

In fact, many companies hoard their users' data. On the Internet, this is known as the "walled garden" effect. Some of the biggest Internet companies on the planet are guilty of this. On Facebook, you cannot export your own data and third parties (like TicTrac) have only limited access to it. Over 2012, Twitter caused an uproar when it began severely curtailing third-party access to its user data. This caused a number of those third parties, who were reliant on Twitter data, to either close down or drastically redesign their services to make use of other data.

So APIs, which enable sharing of user data between applications, are an inherently risky thing for a company like TicTrac. At any time, TicTrac's source of data from companies like Fitbit or Withings could be either cut off or altered. What if Fitbit decided to cut off third-party access to a user's daily steps data, for example? In fact, Fitbit already limits the data it sends out to TicTrac. While I can see my steps data in TicTrac, I cannot view the foods I logged in Fitbit. Essentially then, Fitbit allows third parties to use calories-burned data (steps), but not calories consumed (food). Fitbit does this in order to entice its users to make use of its own website, instead of going to an external service like TicTrac. When you think about it that way, it's a sensible business decision by Fitbit. But it's usually inconvenient for users, not to mention TicTrac.

The other issue that TicTrac has to contend with is errors in the data it does get. I mentioned earlier in the chapter that I encountered some bugs in my early tests of TicTrac when my Fitbit data updated erratically. In effect, I seemed to be missing bits of my Fitbit data—my daily step total on Fitbit.com did not match up with the daily steps total showing on TicTrac. I don't know whose fault that was. Perhaps it was nobody's and the data just got lost somewhere along the way from Fitbit's servers to TicTrac's. Whatever the case, it's further evidence that relying on a third party for data is a risky business. When you consider that even the most technologically advanced Internet company on the planet, Google, couldn't control the ups and downs of third-party applications on its iGoogle product, you begin to get a sense of the challenges for TicTrac.

APIs are a key competitive tool for almost all Internet companies and the big players don't hesitate to exert control over the data that flows into and out of their services. Facebook, the biggest player of them all, has a powerful two-way API. But it limits the data it releases to others and is picky about how it presents third-party data to Facebook users. Hundreds of third-party applications enable their data to display in Facebook. For example, if you use the music streaming service Spotify, the songs you listen to can show up in your Facebook news feed. Facebook calls this "frictionless sharing," because the sharing is automated. You must opt in to this—proving that Facebook did learn a lesson from the Beacon debacle! It's important to note that Spotify has little control over how Facebook users see their Spotify data. At any time Facebook could reduce Spotify's visibility in the news feed. Likewise, Facebook keeps a tight rein on which parts of your user data it lets other services use. You can view *some* of it in TicTrac.

One of TicTrac's default projects is one called "My Facebook." It displays information such as your status updates, checkins, total friends, newest friend, and so on—not all of your Facebook data by any means, but enough to at least make a TicTrac project. Although, as I write this, my Facebook status updates are a month out of date on TicTrac. I don't know whose fault that is, Facebook's or TicTrac's, but that's the risk of APIs in a nutshell.

Wellness, not medicine

TicTrac opened to the public in March 2013. At the time of its public launch, it didn't have any branded or expert projects. But there were a number of projects, created by TicTrac itself, to choose from in the "Project Store." Among them were "Fitness" (including trackers for activity, sleep, and eating), "How I Feel," "My Asthma," and "Digital Life" (tracking your social media usage). You can add, modify, or delete trackers for each of those projects.

TicTrac is primarily targeting consumers, although as mentioned previously it is also partnering with health providers and corporations. While TicTrac has a number of moving parts, mercifully one that is not in its ecosystem is government agencies. That's because TicTrac isn't a medical tool, so it isn't subject to the red tape and regulations that—as we've seen—the personal genomics companies have struggled to contend with. Even if you include data such as blood pressure readings in your TicTrac dashboard, it's not seen as a consumer safety threat by the likes of the FDA. According to Martin Blinder, TicTrac is well and truly on "the wellbeing side of health," rather than the medical side. "We help in prevention through a holistic wellbeing approach," he explained. More marketing speak, but translated it means that TicTrac can avoid the regulations and red tape of the medical establishment. "The second that we get into the more regulated areas of healthcare," said Blinder, "or even devices where you need pre-approval, then you have to start playing a different type of tune." So TicTrac is content to serve the consumer market. That's great news for us consumers, because red tape and regulations often get in the way of looking after your health.

Which brings us to the Electronic Health Record (EHR), the classic example of bureaucracy slowing down technological progress in the health industry. The concept of an EHR is a simple one. No more paper trails across doctors, hospitals, specialists, schools, who knows where else. Instead, your EHR is a single digital file that includes all your health data. However, one of the key problems is that EHRs are still squarely focused on health providers. Many EHRs don't give access to the patient. In hospitals especially, don't expect that to change any time soon. The ideal scenario for EHRs is that you, the consumer, have easy access to your health file as well as your health providers. The file is all about you after all, so why shouldn't you have access to it?

Regardless of who can access it, there have been many attempts to introduce EHR systems into the medical establishment over the years. But it's been a long, slow process. Early EHR systems were PC-based enterprise software suites, deployed in large public hospitals. Thankfully, consumer technology—as it often does—is showing the way forward for EHRs. The iPad was a revolutionary product for the EHR industry, and startups such as drchrono and Practice Fusion were created to build EHRs for the iPad. These developments led to EHRs infiltrating tens of thousands of small-to-medium medical practices. These iPad app EHRs often result in significant time savings to doctors.

In 2012, EHR vendor drchrono surveyed 1,300 US physicians who currently use EHRs. Nearly three-quarters of those physicians said that an EHR has increased the efficiency of their practice. The key efficiency metric, according to a September 2012 interview I carried out with drchrono CEO Michael Nusimow and COO Daniel Kivatonos, is time savings. The report stated that the average time saved using an EHR was 61.7 minutes per day, which is a lot in the busy day of a harried doctor. If any type of EHR has a chance of being accessible to the patient, surely it's an iPad version. Unfortunately, currently even EHR iPad apps aren't very open to consumers. The drchrono report stated that only 10.9% of patients access test results online via their EMR platform. So there is a lot of work to do yet to make truly accessible EHRs a reality among the medical establishment.

Despite the slow progress toward EHRs over the years, since 2009 US adoption has increased, not because of a sudden realization by the medical establishment that digital records are the future, but because of incentives from the US government. A portion of the American Recovery and Reinvestment Act (ARRA), signed in February 2009, was devoted to EHRs. Called the "Health Information Technology for Economic and Clinical Health (HITECH) Act," it provided financial incentives for hospitals and doctors to adopt EHRs. According to the National Center for Health Statistics, 72% of office-based physicians used an electronic medical record or electronic health record (EMR/EHR) system in 2012. That's up from 48% in 2009.

But even with the government's support, there are a number of obstacles that must be overcome before modern EHRs become commonplace in doctors' offices and hospitals. First, an investment in new technology is required. The EHR iPad apps—along with healthy competition among multiple vendors—mean a relatively modest investment for small- to medium-sized medical establishments, such as doctors' offices. But it can be a significant investment for large organizations. A bigger obstacle is changing processes and workflows in medical establishments. That requires a lot of training and changes to how things are done.

That brings us back to TicTrac and its focus on the wellness sector, rather than any attempt to provide a medical service. Essentially this means that TicTrac has far less legwork to do than EHR vendors like drchrono and Practice Fusion. Unlike EHR vendors, TicTrac doesn't have to go through a certification process. Plus it doesn't need to convince the medical establishment to adopt a totally new system, which will be costly and require a significant overhaul of work processes. Compared to EHR vendors, TicTrac has it easy. It can—and indeed did—launch with an incomplete beta service and market itself directly to consumers: you and me. Which we should all be thankful for, since we're still waiting (and waiting …) to get access to our electronic health records. We'll be waiting for a while yet, so we might as well do what we can with our health data on consumer apps like TicTrac. Who knows, one day TicTrac may connect directly to EHRs! But let's not get ahead of ourselves.

Your doctor and you

For consumers, the main benefit of TicTrac (and other emerging health dashboards like it) is that it gives us a tool to track many different data points in one place. If Martin Blinder's big plans come to fruition, TicTrac will also help us make use of that data through insights and expert guidance from nutritionists and the like.

I started this chapter discussing Martin Blinder's trip to his doctor, when he showed the doctor his TicTrac data and graphs. It's important to note that TicTrac—and similar consumer health dashboard tools—are not meant to replace your medical providers. That's a common theme throughout this book. These tools are designed to empower us to track and better manage our own health. They will help us collaborate with our medical providers about our healthcare; they don't replace our doctors. Indeed, if you can point your doctor or specialist to a graph of your daily activity, stress, or anything else you've been tracking about yourself, that data can only help your medical provider understand what your body is going through.

More important, tracking your own body and lifestyle data gives you more control over your own wellbeing—at least compared to someone who relies on their six-month or annual visits to a doctor to track their health status. Plus if TicTrac has anything to do with it, you'll get regular insights and actionable data about your wellbeing.

How do doctors themselves feel about this influx of data from their patients? Let's visit a doctor in New York City to find out ...

CHAPTER NINE

THE MODERN DOCTOR: DR. ROBIN BERZIN

*Health is something you have to deal with yourself. It's
your responsibility. Hopefully we're getting away from the
idea that the doctor hands you health.*

Dr. Robin Berzin, New York City MD

It was August 2006 and 25-year-old Robin Friedlander was at
the New York City studio of XM Satellite Radio, preparing to
meet celebrity doctor Mehmet Oz. She was there to interview
for the position of associate producer on Dr. Oz's new radio
show. The Turkish-American doctor had already made his
mark in television as a regular on the *Oprah Winfrey Show*.
Now he was preparing to establish his brand name on radio.
Friedlander wasn't sure what to expect from Oprah's favorite
doctor. She was not a fan of the *Oprah Winfrey Show* and was
dismissive of daytime TV. After all, she thought indignantly,
she was a college-educated career woman and about to start
medical school! Was this Dr. Oz a quack? But no, she reassured
herself, he was a Professor of Surgery at Columbia University
and an expert in integrative medicine, the type of medicine
she hoped eventually to practice. That's why she applied for
this job. But this Oprah business, she didn't know what to
make of it ...

Robin Friedlander nervously brushed back her long brown
hair and smoothed out her black dress. She looked up just as Dr.

Oz strode out into the foyer to greet her. Tall, with dark wavy hair, he certainly *looked* like a celebrity doctor. He twinkled his brown eyes at Friedlander and reached out to shake her hand. "I read your resume," he said, in a surprising New Jersey accent. "I'm starting a radio show for Oprah," he continued, talking rapidly, "and you're the perfect person for it! You have a journalism background, you're going to medical school and you're interested in integrative medicine—*and* you can write." Friedlander blushed. She was won over.

Integrative medicine

In 2006, Dr. Oz's celebrity career was only just getting going. A few years later he would launch a daytime TV show for Oprah's network, called *The Dr. Oz Show*. Robin Berzin (she married in mid-2013) had big things ahead of her too, having just been accepted into medical school, which she would begin in the New Year. For her pre-med qualification she studied international relations at the University of Pennsylvania. Her first job after graduating in 2003 was as a research coordinator at the NYU School of Medicine. There she'd developed an interest in a style of medicine known as integrative medicine, which had led her to Dr. Oz and his radio show.

Despite Berzin's misgivings about Dr. Oz's celebrity, the job would turn out to be an invaluable introduction to the world of communications technology. She couldn't have known at the time just how important a role technology would play in her future medical career.

Berzin got her chance to practice integrative medicine when she graduated from medical school in 2011. Integrative medicine means incorporating the holistic practices of Eastern medicine into Western medicine, which is very much focused on the physical body. And our doctors are great at diagnosing problems with the body. Where this approach has failed us in the past, and still does, is in preventing those problems from surfacing in the first place. Instead of spending so much time diagnosing sickness, why not spend more time attempting to prevent it?

This is also the key to self-tracking, as explored in this book. Self-tracking is first and foremost a means to *prevent* us from getting sick.

Doctors in the United States "wait until people are sick before they pay attention to them," Robin Berzin told me via a Skype call in 2013. "They often ignore energy levels, relationships, environmental factors, and diet, and lifestyle." As a practicing physician now, Dr. Berzin is keen to put integrative medicine to the test in the real world.

How can integrative medicine help change the US medical system? Well, let's clear up one misconception first. Integrative medicine doesn't necessarily mean that your family doctor needs to bone up on healing crystals or learn how to do acupuncture. What integrative medicine means, to general practitioners like Dr. Berzin, is your doctor collaborating with you to prevent sickness before it occurs, in particular, to make sure you don't come down with the current ailments of the Western world: obesity, type 2 diabetes, and heart disease. This approach requires a more expansive approach to practicing medicine. Not only must your doctor examine your body, but also your mind, the environment you live in, your consumption habits, and your lifestyle. Your doctor can help you prevent heart disease, for example, by encouraging you to reduce your intake of processed foods and to exercise more.

Dr. Oz is one of the leading voices in integrative medicine, although his term for it is "complementary medicine." He uses techniques, such as aromatherapy and meditation, as a complement to traditional Western medicine. An article on his website lists many different forms of complementary medicine: acupuncture, Reiki, massage, chiropractic and osteopathic manipulation, natural products (herbs, omega-3, St. John's wort, and so forth), meditation, diet-based therapies (such as macrobiotic and vegetarian), and relaxing body-mind exercises, such as yoga and t'ai chi. Apart from acting as a celebrity figurehead for all of these complementary medicines, Dr. Oz puts particular emphasis on transcendental meditation in his practice.

Ayurveda: the body as system

Robin Berzin has trained in a few forms of body-mind therapy. She trained (twice) to be a yoga teacher, she has studied meditation, and she trained to be a practitioner of the ancient Indian form of medicine, Ayurveda.

Ayurveda actually means "traditional medicine" in India, although its focus is on channeling energy within the body. Indeed, Ayurveda may be the key to success for integrative medicine in the West, because of its focus on balance. Ayurveda emphasizes the balance of things like food intake, sleep, and sex. Arguably, many of the ills of the Western world are due to imbalances: too much processed food and too little exercise results in diabetes or obesity. So Ayurveda, which seeks a balance of internal and external energies in the body, is an approach worthy of more consideration in Western medicine.

The history of Ayurveda in India goes right back to 3000 BC, in ancient Brahman/Vedic texts describing diseases. By 1500 BC Ayurveda had become a leading—if more magical than medical—method of healing in India. The canonical Sanskrit texts on Ayurveda were written 200 BC and AD 200. They were the medical textbooks of the day and were known as the Charaka Samhita and Sushrita Samhita. The golden age of Ayurveda is considered to be between AD 500–1000, but the influence of this ancient form of medicine is undergoing a renaissance today. Ironically, given its mystical origins, technologists are among the greatest proponents of Ayurveda.

Renowned computer scientist Danny Hillis believes that Ayurvedic theories point to the future of healthcare. A former professor at MIT and a pioneer in supercomputers, Hillis has a formidably logical mind. You might think that a somewhat spiritual theory about medicine has little connection with the high-tech world that Danny Hillis occupies. Yet he has found not only a connection between the two worlds, but also what he thinks is the key to our future wellbeing, which is to treat the body itself as a system in the same way we work with computers and information networks. Taking his cue from Ayurveda, Hillis is approaching medicine with the view that balance is the foundation for good health and imbalance the harbinger of disease.

Hillis' current role is professor of research medicine at USC Keck School of Medicine, where he is busy applying his theory of balance to "proteomics"—the study of proteins in the human body. Using the latest knowledge of proteomics and computing, Hillis and his team are creating models of what a healthy bodily state looks like. The idea is that you will be able to compare your bodily state at any particular time to this model, which Hillis says will enable doctors to treat any imbalances in your body long before the actual symptoms show up. This is preventative medicine at the cutting edge.

Danny Hillis envisions a world where preventative medicine is the norm. The traditional Western medical establishment has followed what Hillis calls a "diagnosis treat paradigm." The goal of most doctors in the United States today is to diagnose problems with your body and then treat them as best they can. That paradigm works well with infectious diseases, which were the primary medical challenge of the 19th century and earlier. But it has failed us in the mid- to late 20th century and beyond, when cancer, heart disease, and autoimmune diseases became society's biggest medical challenges. What all of those have in common, Hillis contends, is that they are what he calls "systems diseases." They have their origins *inside* your body. They're the result of imbalances that have thrown your bodily system out of whack.

The approach Danny Hillis is taking is to measure what your body is doing, via the proteins in your blood cells. This is essentially a much more exact form of self-tracking. If Hillis' experiments succeed, they will revolutionize the way medicine is practiced in the US.

From consultation to collaboration

Proteomics may well alter the medical landscape, but it isn't the only form of technology that is reshaping how medicine is practiced. The way in which doctors communicate with their patients is changing too, in no small part due to technology. This will become ever more important as self-tracking gives the patient an increasing amount of health data—which will need to be communicated somehow to their doctor.

One of the biggest benefits of technology for Robin Berzin, as a young, urban doctor, is that it has opened up the communication lines between her and her patients. Indeed, that's what she admired most about Dr. Mehmet Oz when she began working on his radio show in 2006. Despite radio being an old-fashioned technology, what Dr. Oz was doing with it inspired Berzin to look at other forms of communication. That led her to the Internet technology world, where another kind of revolution was taking place over 2006 and 2007—in social media and personal communications. Smartphones, Facebook, and Twitter were just a few of the innovations of that time. Berzin told me that she saw these tools "as a means of communicating more effectively with more people and fostering behavior change." In particular, she said, she wanted to find out how to use Internet technology to communicate better with her own patients.

Robin Berzin wasn't content with just using technology in the medical world; she wanted to help create it too. In 2011, her fourth and final year of medical school, Berzin and a fellow student started up a company called Cureatr. The startup's name was a mashup of the word "cure" with the social media keyword "curator"—complete with a trendily dropped vowel at the end, inspired by the likes of Flickr and Tumblr. Cureatr was a text messaging and secure communications platform for healthcare providers. Her business partner, Joe Mayer, ultimately left his internship to run the company full-time. But Berzin stayed at school to finish her medical residency. "For me, it was really important to have a clinical role and see patients."

Berzin's interest in social media and online communications stems from her response to one of the main issues the medical establishment has: the perceived paternalistic attitude toward patients. Traditionally, doctors in the West have practiced one-way communication with their patients: do as you're told, because doctor knows best. This superior attitude was reflected in the technology that made its way into the offices of doctors in the 80s and onward. You'd think that when medical records became electronic, which started to happen in the 1980s, it would get easier to share information with patients. But in fact the opposite happened. Electronic medical records were locked up in proprietary IT systems that only doctors and health providers could access. Even now, as I outlined in the previous chapter, the vast majority of patients don't have access to their own electronic medical records.

From a doctor's point of view, while there's still some way to go before medical records are two-way, Berzin told me that the latest IT systems at least free up some of her time. "Technology, for me, is a way to have more time with patients," she explained, "to automate things that need to be automated, like data collection." Dr. Berzin uses an Internet-based Electronic Medical Record (EMR) service from a company called Practice Fusion. Like many modern EMR systems, the one Dr. Berzin uses cannot be accessed by her patients. She makes an effort to share her initial assessment and notes with her patients. But it's a manual process and she is frustrated by it. "I want task lists that my patients and I share," said Berzin. "I want us to share information, because healthcare has to be a collaborative effort."

> "Technology, for me, is a way to have more time with patients."

On the automation side, EMRs have helped Robin Berzin— although she says there's much more they could do. However, when it comes to patient care, Berzin thinks that the modern EMR is not at all helpful. In fact, she says, it's a hindrance. In her residency as a doctor, Berzin found that she was so focused on documentation in the EMR "that I could barely look at the person in front of me." She was also frustrated by the fact she would probably never see that patient again. "They would just get bounced to another one of my co-residents, because that's how residency systems are set up. It's pretty awful. It was hard to even care." She added quickly, "I mean, I cared on a visceral level, but it was hard to be really present because I was so distracted."

Other than EMRs, Berzin believes there is much that can be improved about the way a doctor communicates with her patients. In her view, it's all about creating a trusted relationship with the patient. "I think you have to know this person," she told me earnestly, referring to a typical patient. "You have to believe in them, you have to want to care for them."

The modern doctor-patient relationship, at least as practiced by forward-thinking doctors like Robin Berzin, is more of a collaboration than a consultation. The doctor is still the medical expert, but she is relying on the patient to take more responsibility for their healthcare.

This points to another trend in the medical world: a slow but sure shift from quantity to quality in private doctor practices. I'm sure you've all had the experience of visiting your family doctor, sitting in a waiting room for 30 or more minutes flipping through months-old ratty copies of *People* magazine, then finally being called in by your harried doctor, who proceeds to ask you a few questions, scribbles a prescription for antibiotics and shoves it in your hand, and five minutes later you're standing at the reception desk handing over your Visa card. This "wait and rush" scenario is all too common in doctors' offices. It's not because they don't care for you, it's because they don't have the time to care for you.

You may be wondering how integrative medicine can possibly help when it's asking *more* of doctors, not less. To answer that, let's return to the self-tracking tools that we explored in previous chapters: tools like Fitbit, MyFitnessPal, Withings scale, 23andMe, and uBiome. These and other self-tracking tools help you to measure and monitor various aspects of your health. To see how this will eventually free up doctors' time, we need only look at a group of people who have been self-tracking for decades: diabetics.

Diabetics have long been used to self-monitoring, primarily by testing their blood glucose levels several times a day. I should know, as I'm a type 1 diabetic. Five or six times a day, I do a little prick on my finger with a lancet pen, squeeze a drop of blood onto a test strip and insert the strip into a small electronic meter, which outputs my current blood glucose level. It takes less than a minute each time. However, it wasn't always this easy for diabetics to test their blood sugar levels. Commercial blood sugar meters didn't start coming onto the market until the 1980s, despite prototypes being developed in the late 60s. In fact, prior to 1980, it was *doctors* who carried out blood tests on their diabetic patients.

This state of affairs frustrated one Richard Bernstein, a type 1 diabetic who had been diagnosed way back in 1946, at age twelve. In 1969, Bernstein discovered in a magazine an early prototype for a blood sugar meter. It weighed 3 pounds and cost $650, but was only available to certified physicians and hospitals. Fortunately, Bernstein's wife was a doctor and so he was able to procure the device. His daily blood testing soon helped him gain control over his diabetes, which he later described as a "new sensation of being the boss of my own metabolic state." So enthused with the self-monitoring devices was Richard Bernstein that he attempted to get the medical establishment to prescribe them to their patients. But he was met with a brick wall. He became so frustrated at continual rejection that he felt there was only one course of action left open to him: to become a doctor himself. So he began training to be a doctor in 1979, at age 45!

Richard Bernstein went on to become the most influential doctor in the diabetes field, publishing a landmark book in 1997 called *Dr. Bernstein's Diabetes Solution*. In it he recounts the attitude of the medical establishment in the 1970s toward blood sugar meters: "It was unthinkable that patients be allowed to 'doctor' themselves. They knew nothing of medicine—and if they could, how would doctors earn a living? In those days, patients visited their doctors once a month to 'get a blood sugar.' If they could do it at home for 25 cents (in those days), why pay a physician?"

It's a legitimate question, of course. Why pay a physician? Increasingly, the answer is: because their expertise can help you interpret your data. While it's easy nowadays to monitor various data points about your body, you often still need help interpreting that data. So you have a blood pressure monitoring app for your iPhone. That doesn't necessarily mean you know what the readings mean in relation to your body. But even then, it won't necessarily be physicians who provide that help. Nurses will become better trained to deal with the huge amount of data that self-tracking technology will inevitably output. Which, going back to our original point, frees up doctors like Robin Berzin to spend more quality time with the patients who need their expertise most. Put another way, instead of you going to the doctor four times a year and spending five or ten minutes being rushed through your consultation each time, now you might just see your doctor once a year, but it's a 45-minute consultation—a thorough review of all your personal data and feelings about your health.

From the doctor's point of view, instead of seeing 45 patients for seven minutes each (which is about the norm these days), she will be able to spend 45 minutes each on seven or eight patients per day. This is certainly what Dr. Berzin wants, because it will allow her to truly care for her patients and develop a relationship of mutual trust.

Self-tracking tools: all change is experiential

I wondered whether Dr. Berzin was seeing an increased use among her patients of self-tracking tools, such as the Fitbit activity tracker or the MyFitnessPal food logger. And does she encourage her patients to use these tools, to measure and motivate themselves? "I am seeing more and more of it," she told me. "I wouldn't say it's the norm. Obviously, it skews younger, early adopters. I do encourage it because I think if people like them and it gets them engaged around their health, great. I don't think it's a panacea, but I do think that it gives people a sense of motivation." However, Dr. Berzin is somewhat skeptical of the amount of effort it takes for people to adopt self-tracking tools. Tools like Fitbit and MyFitnessPal "ask people to do a lot," Berzin said. "We in the technology world get really excited about that, but it's a bit blind, I think, to the reality of how hard it is to get people to change how they live every day." Her theory is that people need hands-on help in getting started with these tools, as well as regular encouragement.

"All change is experiential," said Berzin. "You can talk at people till you're blue in the face, you can give them ideas and you can intellectualize. But I think people truly change when something happens to them, when they physically—in person—experience something emotionally salient." To Dr. Berzin, the key to success for the current crop of tools is becoming more user-friendly. Ever since the rise of Steve Jobs, the term "people-centered design" has become a mantra for Internet technology. Jobs and his company Apple helped make personal computers less intimidating for people, less geeky. He did the same for smartphones and then tablets, with the iPhone and iPad. A similar design revolution needs to happen with health applications. One way apps can achieve this is by offering more visualizations of people's data. Dr. Berzin confirmed that this has helped in her practice. "When people see their own data—graphs, charts, and the prettiness factor—that's really important because for people to respond to it, there has to be something emotionally salient there."

Another key is for health applications to be embedded more into technology that we're already using. We've seen the beginning of that revolution, with the rise of smartphone apps, such as the aforementioned blood pressure app. These rely on sensors within the phone, which most of us carry around with us all the time. But increasingly those sensors will be embedded into our clothes or accessories. Eventually that will automate some forms of self-tracking, so that we don't even need to think about them.

That said, a lot of self-tracking will continue to be something we do manually. Certainly much of today's self-tracking requires manual effort. But that's OK, because one thing we've discovered in this book is that you don't need to self-track all the time. Often, tracking something for a month or two is more than sufficient. People use self-tracking inconsistently. This is something that Dr. Berzin has noticed among those of her patients who have tried tools like Fitbit or MyFitnessPal. But as long as the data is useful and there are enough regular measurements to detect trends, then it's helpful to Dr. Berzin's patient care.

Prevention: health is on you

Like Danny Hillis, and all the gurus, Dr. Berzin's true passion as a doctor is prevention. She'd rather not just intervene when a person is already sick, but help that person prevent sickness from occurring in the first place. "I'm really interested in galvanizing people to change their behavior, to be proactive." One of Dr. Berzin's catchphrases is "health is on you." She strongly believes that "health is something you have to deal with yourself. It's your responsibility. Hopefully we're getting away from the idea that the doctor hands you health."

This isn't a new idea, taking responsibility for your own health. Indeed, it's been a maxim of many doctors over the years. The trouble is, a lot of those doctors have been seen as renegades—or worse, as quacks. A notable example from my own country, New Zealand, is one Dr. Ulric Williams. Born in 1890, he went to the UK and trained to be a doctor at Cambridge and Edinburgh Universities.

> "I'm really interested in galvanizing people to change their behavior, to be proactive."

He returned to New Zealand, becoming a family doctor and hospital surgeon in a small North Island city called Wanganui. From his beginnings as a practicing physician in 1918, Dr. Williams developed a reputation as a playboy. However, in his late thirties, he had a religious conversion and began railing against the orthodox medical establishment. In a strange mix of religious-speak and alternative medicine mumbo-jumbo, Dr. Williams wrote a book entitled *Hints on Healthy Living* in 1934. Despite the mild title, the writing inside the book is brash and highly opinionated. Here's the opening couple of sentences from the foreword to the first edition:

It can no longer be denied that the GREAT cause of
sickness is disobedience to natural law—wrong manner
of living. A very large proportion of disease from which
mankind suffers is IMMEDIATELY PREVENTABLE.

The all-capitals words are from Dr. Williams. He makes continuous use of capital letters throughout his book and other things he would go on to write, including a 1941 pamphlet entitled "Hospitals and hooey or health?" His eccentricity and contemptuous attitude toward the medical establishment made him a standout character in the otherwise staid, conservative New Zealand culture of the 1940s and 50s. But his outrageous manner also made it easy for the medical powers to dismiss him as a quack. However, if you look behind the pompous capitalization and guilt-inducing religious rhetoric ("disobedience," "wrong," "suffers"), Dr. Williams' core message is one that American self-help pioneer Ralph Waldo Emerson himself would have applauded: take responsibility for your own health. "Reform begins with the individual," Dr. Williams wrote in *Hints on Healthy Living.*

Dr. Williams' book recommends taking stock of your lifestyle habits, including what you eat and drink. In the foreword to the third edition of the book, he wrote: "We have conceived of disease as something attacking us from without, due to germs; whereas disease, whether of body, mind, soul or estate, is mostly a gradual degenerative process going on within, due to failure to comply with the requirements of well-being."

This idea that sickness comes with within, rather than without, is echoed today by people like Danny Hillis. And medically speaking, it's undeniably true. The diseases of today are things that happen within our bodies: cancer, autoimmune diseases, heart disease—what Danny Hillis calls "systems diseases," with the system in this case being our own body.

Some of what Dr. Williams wrote has not stood the test of time. For example, his ludicrously moralistic stance on cancer— "psychological turmoil" and "wrong thinking," he puffed, can lead to cancer. Nevertheless, Dr. Williams' core principles about health are sound: what you eat and how you live are key causes of disease in the human body.

The main difference between Dr. Williams' era and the present day has been the rise of tools that help people help themselves. But that doesn't mean it's any less confusing for the average person. Dr. Berzin acknowledges that even in this day and age, there is anxiety and fear around people taking more responsibility for their own health. People want to know exactly how they do this. They're confused about these new-fangled tools like Fitbit and MyFitnessPal. "There's a lot of chaos," Dr. Berzin told me. "There are a lot of tools. And yet, this is the first time we've been able to manage, control, and interact with our data to understand ourselves a little bit better." For Dr. Berzin, it all comes back to the patient. Sometimes the latest technology isn't the answer—at least in the beginning. "You have to know your patient," she asserted. "I have patients for whom offering an activity tracker is like offering them a trip to Mars. It's just not going to be a salient, meaningful thing that they can incorporate into their lives. You really have to meet people where they are."

I asked Dr. Berzin how she would approach a patient who came to her overweight and was clearly at risk of developing type 2 diabetes, the most common form of diabetes and the one associated with excess weight. One approach she would take, she replied, is to help the patient achieve incremental change by reinforcing and measuring what they are already doing. "So if somebody is already an exerciser," said Berzin, "but they're not doing quite enough of it, I'll offer them a plan to help motivate them." For example, she'd encourage the patient to enroll in a gym program. This is fairly common advice to overweight people, from doctors and indeed from family and friends around them. But the thing is, diet and exercise can actually cure a type 2 diabetic.

When you hear the word "cure," you probably typically think of a medical solution—drugs via a prescription from your doctor, or surgery. But integrative medicine as practiced by Dr. Berzin and many other modern doctors takes a much broader view of curing a patient. Let's look at type 2 diabetes, as it's a great example of what can be done outside drugs and surgery.

Type 2 diabetes is not a disease, it's a metabolic disorder. It's when the body can no longer process insulin efficiently, which means that blood sugar levels become elevated. This is often referred to as "insulin resistance," because the body fails to deal with insulin the way it's supposed to. Type 2 is closely associated with obesity, because when the body gains excess weight it can sometimes lead to problems regulating blood glucose. However, it's important to note that not all type 2 diabetics are obese, or even overweight. It can be caused by a genetic malfunction, for example the liver not processing glucose properly. Also, non-obese women are more prone to type 2 diabetes.

Type 2 makes up 85–90% of the total number of cases of diabetes. But it is in fact entirely different from type 1, which is an autoimmune disease. The only thing the two types have in common is the main symptom: high blood glucose levels. However, type 2 patients can still produce insulin, whereas in type 1 the pancreas no longer produces insulin (or, in less severe cases, isn't producing enough of it). This effectively means that while type 1 cannot be cured at this time, type 2 can be. What is the type 2 cure? Well, drugs can and do help; but in most cases the patient can cure themselves through diet and exercise alone. Making adjustments to the patient's eating and exercise habits helps the body regulate insulin properly again.

Craig Bell is a 61-year-old from Oregon. He not only suffered from type 2 diabetes, but fibromyalgia (chronic pain), and depression too. He is adamant that personal responsibility was the key to curing his type 2, not treatment by a doctor. Bell was diagnosed with type 2 in 2003, at age 51. Initially he was prescribed a drug called Metformin, a very common drug for type 2. But not only did it not help, he actually gained weight and his blood glucose levels kept creeping up. At 5 foot 11 inches, Bell weighed 215 pounds a couple of years after his diagnosis. Frustrated, he stopped taking Metformin at that point and embarked on a new diet and exercise regime. The diet was "nutrient-rich, low glycemic index, natural foods based." He supplemented this with walking "at least an hour and a half" every day. "I keep up with many joggers," he told me proudly. By the summer of 2008, Bell's weight had dropped to 172 pounds. He'd effectively cured himself of type 2, without the use of drugs or surgery.

The point isn't that type 2 drugs can't help—in many cases they do. The point is that by taking responsibility for your healthcare, which usually means altering your diet and becoming more active, you can prevent or cure a condition such as type 2 diabetes. If you had a choice between taking drugs for the rest of your life to keep a health condition under control, or taking more responsibility for your own body through diet and exercise, which would you choose?

A common retort to this advice is: easier said than done! It didn't work for me, say many type 2 diabetics. Indeed that is a problem. It is true that eating better and doing more exercise is much harder for some people than it was for Craig Bell. Dr. Berzin often comes across such people and her remedy is complementary therapies. "Sometimes the reasons that people get to a place where they're really overweight and not taking care of themselves go deeper," she told me, "even when they are incredibly effective in their jobs, hard working, and organized in the rest of their lives." In these cases Dr. Berzin tries to get beyond the weight readings and coax her patient to take responsibility for their body. She finds that yoga and meditation help people become more aware of their bodies. "I tend to find that I work with those people a lot with yoga, because it helps them *feel* their bodies," she said. "It's almost like they're not even aware of the fact that they're overweight, yet they have a metabolic syndrome that's going to lead to type 2 diabetes in ten years. It's completely preventable."

It's not all touchy-feely medicine. Yoga may actually have clinical benefits to type 2 diabetics, although so far there is only limited research to back that up. A research paper published in 2010 by three students at the Universities of Ottawa and Toronto, in Canada, showed that yoga can be beneficial to people with type 2 diabetes. While it stopped short of making a specific recommendation for physicians, the study showed "a general beneficial effect of yoga on diabetic patients." Those benefits included better fasting plasma glucose (FPG) levels and lipid profiles—two key markers of health for diabetics, measuring blood sugar level and the health of cells respectively. The report concluded that there were favorable short-term effects of yoga on type 2 diabetics, although there was no proof of favorable long-term outcomes.

Prescribing apps

We've seen in this chapter that technology has been an important aspect of Dr. Robin Berzin's medical training, and now practice— at first, as a way to enhance communication with her patients, and later through consumer devices and apps that people can use to monitor their own health. Yet above all, Dr. Berzin wants to do what's best for her patients. Sometimes that might be prescribing a Fitbit device for a patient who is in danger of developing type 2 diabetes. Other times she would find it more appropriate to prescribe a course of yoga, or a gym membership, or a combination of those things with drug treatment. It all comes back to the patient and what is appropriate for them and what they would be comfortable trying.

In short, Dr. Berzin collaborates with her patients to find out what would work best for them. She then draws up a plan for the patient to carry out. That's a very different model from the old, paternalistic doctor-patient relationship, where the doctor might scribble a prescription for weight-loss pills and wish the patient good luck.

Doctors today are increasingly open to prescribing consumer technology, but only if it suits the patient and is clinically relevant. Another relatively new doctor, Dr. Jae Won Joh from Houston, Texas, believes that a health technology product must be "clinically compelling" for him to prescribe it to a patient. Dr. Joh's specialty is emergency medicine and he is skeptical, for example, about apps that measure your heart rate. "Clinically, I couldn't care less, and I don't think the vast majority of patients should either. Anyone can get their heart rate in fifteen seconds for free by putting two fingers on their wrist/neck while looking at a clock and doing some basic math." Having said that, he is confident that other apps do provide what he calls "meaningful health benefits in realistic scenarios." He listed the Withings scale, the RunKeeper app, and Sanofi's iBGStar device as current examples of apps he would have no hesitation in prescribing, if the patient might benefit from it.

Of course, because these are consumer-oriented devices and apps, you don't even need a prescription to use them. You only need to place an order on a website or download a new app from the App Store. Increasingly, you won't see your doctor as a conduit to treatment, a paternalistic figure who tells you what you need and who has control over your treatment. Instead you'll view your doctor as a partner in your overall treatment plan—a medical expert who helps guide you to the tools and drugs you need, and helps you interpret your health data.

The other significant change to the doctor-patient relationship that we've explored in this chapter is that it's becoming more focused on preventing sickness, rather than treating symptoms. Again, consumer health technology is playing a key role in this shift, alongside integrative medicine therapies such as yoga.

If there is one overriding theme to the new doctor-patient relationship as practiced by Dr. Berzin in New York City, it's that the patient has much more responsibility for their own health now. As Dr. Berzin likes to say, your health is on you.

CHAPTER TEN

TRACKING + MEDICINE: MD REVOLUTION

In the last year, I've learned more about how to be healthy than I've done in the previous 17 years. And it's because I learned to measure things.

Dr. Samir Damani, cardiologist and founder of MD Revolution

In a previous chapter we looked at a health dashboard called TicTrac. We discovered that it's a free Internet tool that anyone can use, much like Google's search engine or Yahoo's Web email. In this chapter we look at a different kind of dashboard. While it's not free, it has something that TicTrac does not: a medical pedigree. The product is called RevUp and it was created by a cardiologist from San Diego, Dr. Samir Damani.

Dr. Damani's company, MD Revolution, is part dashboard and part medical advice service. Like TicTrac, it's an online dashboard where you can aggregate data from a variety of health tracking tools—Fitbit, Withings scale, MyFitnessPal, and more. You can access this dashboard on the Web and on your smartphone. Also like TicTrac, MD Revolution helps you interpret the data. But this is where their approaches differ. As we saw, TicTrac has set up a marketplace where trained healthcare providers—like nutritionists and personal trainers—compete to offer their services to you. With MD Revolution, you'll also get access to nutritionists, personal trainers, and other healthcare providers. However, you will pay directly for it (or the company you work for will). It's a straight payment-for-services-rendered equation; MD Revolution is selling you its medical expertise.

MD Revolution's office is close by the Scripps Memorial Hospital in La Jolla, just outside San Diego. The location is no coincidence because much of Dr. Samir Damani's medical career has been spent at the Scripps institution. After graduating from the Medical College of Georgia as a doctor in 2003, he started his residency at Scripps Clinic in 2006. He went on to develop expertise in the areas of cardiovascular disease and internal medicine, eventually completing a masters in clinical investigation at the Scripps Research Institute.

It was at Scripps that Damani first became interested in digital health. His biggest influence was another Scripps doctor, who was one of the leading voices in digital health: Dr. Eric Topol. Also a cardiologist, Dr. Topol published a book called *The Creative Destruction of Medicine* in 2012. He even promoted it on the *Stephen Colbert Show*, giving digital health a boost in the mainstream media. Dr. Damani published research papers with Dr. Topol while the two worked together at Scripps, mostly on the medical application of genomics. It was during this period that Dr. Damani began to recommend digital health devices to his patients.

In a phone call in mid-2013, Dr. Damani explained to me the genesis of MD Revolution. "In my clinical practice," he told me, "I'd give my patients weight scales or blood pressure monitors. I would manage them and they would be more engaged in their health. Yet there was no ecosystem." In short, Dr. Damani was impressed by the number of health tracking devices coming out—such as the Fitbit and MyFitnessPal—but he felt there was no easy way for his patients to interpret the data from those devices. "What I realized," he told me, "was that you have to build a model around the delivery of these tools. A model which shows how these tools interact with each other. You need to help people understand what that data means."

So Dr. Damani set out to build a platform that would help his patients make sense of information gathered from services like Fitbit and 23andMe. He raised money and developed the software in 2012. That same year, MD Revolution launched and began to test the service on patients.

It's about the outcomes

MD Revolution is very early in its life as I write this. But essentially what it's selling is a "personalized health program" that utilizes both self-tracking tools (like Fitbit) and genomic information from 23andMe. Dr. Damani's catchphrase for MD Revolution is: "Measure, Monitor, Motivate."

The first thing that happens when you sign up to MD Revolution is a "welcome assessment," which can be done online or at MD Revolution's La Jolla lab. In the initial assessment, you're put through a series of biometric tests to determine your resting metabolic rate, cardiovascular fitness, and other health indicators. This is followed by a medical exam with one of MD Revolution's clinicians, who also schedules lab tests for you. A few days after the first assessment, you have a consultation with an MD Revolution nutritionist. In this session your current diet and eating habits are analyzed, from which a personal diet plan is created. A day or two after that, you attend a "Fitness & Digital Health Session," in which you're assisted with the setup of tracking devices and smartphone apps.

> Dr. Damani's catchphrase for MD Revolution is: "Measure, Monitor, Motivate."

At the time of writing, MD Revolution partners with four tracking services: Fitbit (activity tracker), Withings (scale), Digifit (heart rate monitor), and MyFitnessPal (food tracking). All of these products are connected into the MD Revolution dashboard, called RevUp. You're given an account in RevUp and shown how to use it. As well as the digital integration, this final session gives you a personalized exercise program, so you know exactly what you'll be tracking. Finally, if you haven't already done a DNA test, then MD Revolution will organize this for you.

MD Revolution has a team of specialists who you will meet, whether in the flesh or virtually, in the first week. The core members of the team are a nutritionist, a personal trainer, and a "health coach." After the initial exam and these specialist consultations, most of MD Revolution's service is virtual. You're offered feedback and guidance by the various specialists via the website, which happens about once a fortnight. If a clinical consultation is needed, more often than not it's done via Skype. But typically, says Dr. Damani, no further consultations are necessary after the initial exam. "What we do is monitor and motivate," Dr. Damani told me. "All of that can be done virtually. And we literally have people all over the world who have come in, done their initial assessments, and then we just monitor and motivate them. They do the measuring and we help with the collection. We do the interpreting and explaining, but all that is virtual."

The entire MD Revolution program typically lasts a whole year. But the first three months are key and the most intense. The initial assessment and setup of devices and apps is all done in the first couple of weeks. After a month, you check in to see whether the program is going smoothly. This includes a review of your exercise program and its attendant fitness apps, a metabolic reassessment done six weeks after the initial tests, and a review of your genetics results. After twelve weeks in the program, you're given the option of doing a full reassessment of all tests. These various health and fitness tests are a mix of clinical tests (the same as those your own doctor does for you from time to time) and the type of assessment you would undergo if you joined a gym. But the clinical tests are really the crucial part. MD Revolution is, after all, a medical service.

While signing up to MD Revolution is akin to going for an annual medical checkup with your doctor, you may have noticed that two words have been conspicuously absent from this chapter so far. Those words, "prescription" and "drugs," have become synonymous with going to a doctor. But although MD Revolution's service does include a consultation with a clinician—sometimes Dr. Damani himself, a practicing cardiologist—the focus isn't on prescribing drugs to treat a condition or disease. Instead it's about making subtle changes to your daily diet and exercise routines in order to prevent disease, or (in the case of existing chronic conditions such as type 2 diabetes) achieving what Dr. Damani repeatedly refers to as "outcomes."

The outcomes that MD Revolution puts the most emphasis on are a healthy heart and optimal body fat level. One of the markers that MD Revolution measures is VO2, which is the body's ability to consume oxygen. According to MD Revolution's website, VO2 is "the best measure of cardiorespiratory fitness." VO2, along with measurements such as body fat, resting metabolic rate, and trunk fat, are the key metrics of success for an MD Revolution customer.

One of the most important things MD Revolution is doing is putting in context the information people can gather from using free tools like Fitbit and MyFitnessPal. It's all very well walking 10,000 steps a day or eating less than 100 grams of carbohydrates per day, but what you really want to know—and understand—is how that is impacting your daily health. Through VO2, body fat, and other measurements, MD Revolution helps you monitor the actual changes in your body. The Fitbit information you see in your RevUp dashboard is actually the same information you'd see on Fitbit's website—often less, because Fitbit doesn't allow all of its user data to be seen in external apps. But crucially, MD Revolution combines that Fitbit data with other pieces of data in order to help you better understand it. You see your average heart rate, for example. This data comes from another device, DigiFit.

Your fitness-related genetics are also displayed on RevUp, on the same page as your Fitbit data. For example, if your DNA shows that you have enhanced insulin sensitivity response to regular exercise, then this information is displayed as motivation to exercise. RevUp also adds its own custom graphics for Fitbit data, such as a bar chart for daily steps and a pie chart for how much of your daily exercise was "very active," "fairly active," "lightly active," and "sedentary." That information comes from Fitbit itself, but RevUp makes it slightly prettier and easier to digest.

Finally, RevUp uses a points system to interpret your Fitbit data into more readily understood terms. If you have a daily step goal of 7,000, for example, and you do 8,000 steps on a particular day, you might get five points. But if you do just 2,000 steps, you might only get one point. The points system isn't set in stone; it's customized for you at the start of the program. It's the same type of gamification that Buster Benson (in Chapter One) uses in his custom-designed self-tracking apps. The points in RevUp add a game element to your MD Revolution program, which may be useful if you're a competitive type of person who is motivated by chasing points. According to the company, the points also correlate with real health outcomes.

Like going to the gym

Dr. Damani sees his startup as being a new specialty in medicine, in other words, a specialized service that doctors can refer their patients to when necessary. He believes that doctors have neither the time nor the technical inclination to prescribe their patients self-tracking devices. "They don't have time to help with prevention and nutritional counseling," said Dr. Damani about his fellow physicians. "They don't have time to teach people how to use these devices. They don't have an IT person in their practice to tell a patient how to use MyFitnessPal. They don't have people to show them how to set up a Withings scale at their house, or how to integrate 23andMe. And most doctors don't know how to use genetic information in their practices."

As we saw with Dr. Robin Berzin in the previous chapter, there's no doubt that doctors are pressed for time. They're too busy treating patients who are already well past the prevention stage. But what if doctors could refer their regular patients to a service that can assist with prevention and nutrition? According to Dr. Damani, MD Revolution is stepping up to fill this gap. The macro level view is that the more people improve their daily health, the less likely they are to get sick— and so the less pressure on doctors over time, which in turn, one hopes, will allow doctors to focus back on prevention. Most people in the medical establishment agree that this is the ideal long-term outcome for healthcare. The question is how to get there. At the very least, MD Revolution takes some of the prevention workload off doctors in the short term. In fact MD Revolution is already getting referrals from doctors, says Dr. Damani. "Our biggest referrals are from primary care physicians," he told me in mid-2013. I asked if the data from MD Revolution is shared with the patient's doctor. "All the data is shared back with them," Dr. Damani assured me.

MD Revolution does indeed seem to be a new type of healthcare service. To help promote this new paradigm, Dr. Damani offers up an interesting comparison between MD Revolution and gyms. Both rely on subscriptions to make their money. From the customer's point of view, you pay MD Revolution a subscription every month for a service that improves your health, just as you do with a gym membership. It can cost as little as $5 per month for a limited MD Revolution membership (for access to the dashboard only), going up to $60 per month for a full-service membership. And the more of their employees they sign up, the lower the rates become for corporations. This is similar to how gyms work, with varying tiers of monthly membership and incentives for corporations.

Dr. Damani reiterated that MD Revolution is not in the business of making hardware devices, so it won't be competing with the likes of Fitbit or Withings. "We're device agnostic," he declared. "We are in the game of showing people how to use these devices to better their health." In a way, that's similar to how gyms make their money by supplying the hardware (treadmills, exercycles, crosstrainers, weights, and bars) and then showing you how to use it. Gyms often help you customize an exercise program to suit your needs, show you how to use the equipment, set certain weight or fitness goals for you, and so on. While MD Revolution doesn't pay for the devices it prescribes—you have to buy your own Fitbit or Withings scale—it does teach you how to use them and helps you interpret the data.

To stretch the comparison a bit further, a gym is also a kind of "ecosystem" of fitness equipment. A treadmill is a means of helping you walk more steps, with varying levels of resistance applied to help tone your leg muscles. A barbell has a completely different purpose, to help build muscle in your forearms and shoulders. But the treadmill and the barbell—along with the many other pieces of equipment in a typical gym—complement each other and belong together under one roof. Likewise, a Fitbit has a different purpose than, say, a heart monitor device. MD Revolution brings together these and other self-tracking devices (or at least the best-of-breed ones) into a single ecosystem. Each device has a specific purpose, but they work together to provide a full picture of a person's health.

RevUp

Healthcare guidance is primarily what you're subscribing to with MD Revolution, but the core of its service is the online dashboard product. Called RevUp, as noted earlier, it's similar to TicTrac in that it aggregates data from various tracking devices. So you can track your Fitbit data in RevUp, alongside other services such as the Withings scale and MyFitnessPal.

RevUp is organized into the following categories: Health (your health markers such as weight, body fat, blood pressure); Nutrition (including information from MyFitnessPal, if you use that app); Fitness (Fitbit and the like); Genetics; Challenges. That last category is for health goals, such as running a marathon. What's immediately noticeable about RevUp is how it utilizes graphs and the now familiar thumbs-up/thumbs-down icons to make your health data easier to scan and digest. It's almost like a Facebook for health data. RevUp also has automated software that monitors your data. So, for example, if your set goal is 10,000 steps per day and you haven't hit that goal in a few days, then MD Revolution's staff get a message and they can then nudge you via text or email.

According to Dr. Damani, MD Revolution's users are more motivated to work on their health if they have clear guidance about what the various data points signify—and what they can do to improve that data. "For example," explained Dr. Damani, "if you have a high risk for diabetes type 2, that information is right next to your step calendar and your weight." RevUp makes use of graphics and colors to emphasize risks. In this case, your high risk of getting type 2 diabetes is indicated by the information being colored bright red and having an ominous-looking thumbs-down icon next to your reading. "Patients know it's probabilistic," he continued, "so it's not like they're necessarily going to develop it. But they're much more motivated, because there's clear guidance on what they can do about it."

It all comes down to behavioral science, says Dr. Damani. "What we have are clearly delineated steps for people based on them looking at their own data. When you start looking at your own data, it's really easy to enhance or change your behavior. Because all of a sudden, it's in your face."

One area where MD Revolution is noticeably different from TicTrac is in its integration of genomic information. Part of the initial consultation with MD Revolution involves doing a DNA test, which the company does in association with its partner 23andMe. The real value-add comes in how MD Revolution utilizes the resulting genetic data in its health monitoring service. But how are they doing this, when (as we've seen in previous chapters) most of the medical establishment still doesn't know how to make use of genetic data in healthcare?

Dr. Damani agreed that so far personal genomics services like 23andMe have fallen short of high expectations: "The problem is that these genetic reports are probabilistic, they're not deterministic. Basically, it's no different from stepping on a scale if you're obese and then saying 'I have a risk for diabetes.' It doesn't mean you're going to develop it. So the problem with the current model, just disseminating genetic data, is that it doesn't give you clear action items.

"I don't believe in just throwing everything out there," said Dr. Damani said of genetic information. "I think 23andMe is wonderful, but the problem is they're not clinicians. Their expertise has been getting it to the consumers and getting them engaged. Our job is outcomes." Because MD Revolution is focused on health outcomes, it is very selective about which genotype data it uses. "We have to strategically pick variants and conditions that we think are relevant," said Dr. Damani. "The things that can be changed, or something done about, or to increase awareness on behalf of the patient."

As well as being selective, MD Revolution attempts to match up your genetic data with aspects of your nutrition and daily activity. "So it might be that you're more prone to Vitamin D deficiency," Dr. Damani said. "Well now, on your nutrition page you'll see that you're more prone to Vitamin D deficiency." That motivates you to eat more Vitamin D foods and also allows you—and the MD Revolution team—to monitor this over time.

The technical term for information about your daily nutrition and activity is "phenotypes." We first came across this word in the chapter about 23andMe. There we met the startup Curious, which is trying to merge genotype with phenotype data by asking people to upload their 23andMe results and at the same time answer various questions about their daily health habits. By filling in surveys about their food and exercise habits, 23andMe itself is trying to get more people to enter their phenotype information. MD Revolution thinks it has the edge though, because it's coming at the issue from a clinical perspective and is integrating real-time measuring tools like Fitbit and MyFitnessPal. "For the first time," said Dr. Damani, "genetic data will be able to yield insights to phenotypes that fall within our system." He means that MD Revolution will combine the patient's genetic data with all of the other collected data in the RevUp dashboard.

If MD Revolution is able to successfully make use of genetic data now, then this has long-term benefits too. "A few years from now," said Dr. Damani, "we're going to be able to see, for example, what the obesity variance is." This is the genetic marker that shows an increased risk of developing obesity. "How does that," he continued, "impact on the ability of people to lose weight, using digital health tools like a heart rate monitor or a Fitbit? How do steps correlate with the reduction of fat, versus performing interval training using a heart rate monitor?" Dr. Damani is convinced that this merging of genetic and phenotypic data is the next step in personal genomics.

Ultimately it's about us, the consumers. How do we make use of our DNA data to improve our day-to-day health? Dr. Damani believes he can provide "a clear path for the patient," in the form of RevUp and his healthcare providers who give guidance. With MD Revolution, he concluded, "your genetic data is placed in context of creating a health picture for you."

Compliance and behavior change

Back in the TicTrac chapter, I mentioned that TicTrac isn't promoting itself as a medical system and therefore doesn't need to be compliant with US health regulations, in particular the set of HIPAA regulations for healthcare services. HIPAA stands for Health Insurance Portability and Accountability Act, which is administered by the US Department of Health and Human Services. While the emphasis is on health insurance, a key goal of the Act is to ensure the privacy and safety of patients in the healthcare system.

Unlike TicTrac, MD Revolution *is* promoting itself as a medical service. Indeed, in its FAQs MD Revolution describes itself as a "physician practice" and "completely HIPAA-compliant." Despite the red tape associated with government compliance, one big benefit is that MD Revolution's IT system can more easily interface with other healthcare providers. That's because HIPAA includes a set of computing standards. Dr. Damani mentions Electronic Health Record (EHR) systems in particular. As noted in the TicTrac chapter, EHRs are increasingly being adopted in physician practices across the US, thanks in large part to a major amendment to the HIPAA regulations in 2009. That was when the US Congress passed the Health Information Technology for Economic and Clinical Health Act (HITECH), which added a technology focus to HIPAA. One of the key provisions of that Act was the incentivization of physician practices to implement electronic health records.

If MD Revolution is indeed a physician practice, then the equivalent of an EHR system for its practice is RevUp, the company's dashboard for health and fitness data. Dr. Damani pointed out that RevUp is "written in a code that can be attached to any existing electronic medical records system." So, he said, a popular EHR like Practice Fusion can "talk to RevUp, or RevUp can talk to it." Dr. Damani thinks that HIPAA compliance will ultimately benefit doctors because they can tap into MD Revolution to help their patients get healthier. "So any doctor who wants to be more proactive with a patient in terms of behavior modification is able to use our platform." So-called wellness services like TicTrac don't need to comply with HIPAA, so they may have the edge in short-term adoption by consumers. But perhaps in the long run it will be consumer services that directly interface with IT systems in hospitals and doctor practices which have the advantage. MD Revolution is banking on this.

One of the criticisms of the HIPAA regulations is that they still have doctors at the center of the ecosystem in terms of patient data. With most EHRs, even the modern technology-focused ones like Practice Fusion, the data is still input—and thus essentially owned—by the physician practice or hospital. So you go to your doctor, and it's the doctor's notes that are entered into the EHR system. Even if you brought along your Fitbit or MyFitnessPal data, it's unlikely to be entered into the EHR. What's more, many EHRs nowadays don't give the patient access to their own data. However, MD Revolution may be the bridge to a more patient-centered ecosystem for electronic health records. Both healthcare provider and patient enter data into RevUp. And, crucially, the patient always has access to their health information.

The next step, after the patient gaining control of their own data, is to enable the wider sharing of health data to improve healthcare across a whole country. Data sharing, in an anonymous way so that patient privacy isn't compromised, is a growing grassroots movement in the healthcare industry. The reason why this is important is that more open sharing of health data will lead to further insights in so-called population health management. In other words, understanding the health of an entire country's population will, in turn, lead to more medical breakthroughs. But first things first: let's get electronic health records into the hands of the patient before we start sharing them around. MD Revolution is playing its part there.

Of course, you don't need to sign up to a gym to stay active. You can simply go for a 30-minute walk every day. If you want to measure it, you can attach a Fitbit to your body. Or if you want to build muscle, there are various exercises you can do at home: push-ups, sit-ups, jogging on the spot. You can enter each day's exercise into Fitbit's portal, or for that matter in a paper journal. In short, of the three elements in MD Revolution's mantra—"Measure, Monitor, Motivate"—you can do a good enough job of the first two on your own. It seems to me that the key aspect of MD Revolution's offering is the third part: motivation. Many of us are good at starting a new exercise routine, but it's pushing on with it when it becomes a chore that is the problem. When you have a team of healthcare professionals guiding you, and you're paying them, then the motivation is clear.

This may be the biggest problem of the first wave of self-tracking companies, like Fitbit and MyFitnessPal. Each of those two companies offers a product. In the case of Fitbit, it's a tracking device and a website to view your data from that device. In the case of MyFitnessPal, it's a software app that enables you to track your food input every day. But the motivation aspect of self-tracking falls purely on you, the consumer. And as we saw in the first chapter about uber self-tracker Buster Benson, motivating yourself to improve or change is a very tough thing to do on your own. It all comes down to behavior change, which is hard graft any way you look at it. Buster Benson struggles with changing his behaviors to this day, perhaps because he tries to do everything on his own. This is why organizations like Weight Watchers, which we profiled in Chapter Four, are so successful. Their number-one feature is a social support system for behavior change to help you get through the tough times.

Dr. Damani thinks he's found an alternative to the social support system of behavior change so well deployed by Weight Watchers. His solution relies more on medical expertise than group dynamics. Nobody is more of an expert on your health than your family doctor. Then again, nobody knows more about your own body than you. So Dr. Damani's solution is to provide a link between the two. MD Revolution is essentially a middle layer between self-tracking devices (like Fitbit and MyFitnessPal) and your doctor.

Dr. Damani thinks this will lead to a change in the way we think of doctors. Our current health paradigm is that you only go to your doctor when you're sick. Dr. Damani calls this a "reactive model of medicine." With MD Revolution, he is pushing for "a proactive form of medicine that emphasizes prevention." Doctors simply don't have time to regularly motivate you to care for your health, so it will be services like MD Revolution which fill that gap. The tools, says Dr. Damani, aren't enough by themselves. Behavior change only comes about when you have support—whether from peers, or from the medical fraternity. MD Revolution wants to be your medical support system.

> **MD Revolution is essentially a middle layer between self-tracking devices and your doctor.**

Corporate motivation

If MD Revolution had to rely on individual memberships to make money, it would struggle—certainly in this era when doctors are still largely practicing so-called reactive medicine. MD Revolution's solution is to get corporations to sign up their employees en masse. This has big ramifications not only for the future of healthcare, but for patient privacy.

Dr. Damani uses the term "workforce wellness" to describe efforts by corporations to help their employees adopt healthy lifestyles. The economic benefit to corporations is clear: the healthier your employees are, the fewer sick days they take, leading to lower health insurance premiums over time, which also lead to increased productivity, plus of course the bottom line, increased profitability. An MD Revolution white paper cites "dozens of studies" that "demonstrate an average $3 for every $1 return on investment (ROI) from corporate wellness programs." What's more, states the white paper, "that ROI grows to six to one if just 10% of those at high risk (those with two or more chronic disease risk factors) can be moved to lower risk profiles."

However, the problem isn't just signing up corporations to wellness programs, but motivating the employees to follow through. The white paper cites a report by the Institute of Medicine, "Healthy People 2010," which states that "participation in programs is poor with the most motivated individuals participating, and those with greatest potential benefit opting out." Going back to my point about motivation being a key ingredient in MD Revolution's service, this is where Dr. Damani believes his company is poised to make a big impact. The current health system is not only reactive, it also reacts far too slowly. In addition, it fails to give patients the tools to improve their own health. In stark contrast, MD Revolution is, according to its own white paper, offering "a dynamic model that leverages self-tracking."

Dr. Damani told me that there are three different interfaces to RevUp, the health and fitness dashboard. First is the individual patient dashboard, which I've described in the course of this chapter. The second is a special view for MD Revolution's clinical team, which enables them to monitor multiple patients and set up alerts. The third is a dashboard designed for corporations. In Dr. Damani's words, this "outlines the entire population." In other words, a corporation can monitor the health of all its employees in the system. "For example," continued Dr. Damani, "for the first time you'll be able to see how many fit days your patient [i.e. the employee] has, you'll be able to see how many pounds of fat they lost, how many minutes of exercise they did, what is their average heart rate, what is their average BMI." He added that all of this information is anonymized so corporations cannot identify an individual. That's part of the HIPAA regulations, to protect patient privacy. Even so, there is an obvious danger that an employee's "wellness"—or lack thereof—could be used against them.

As self-tracking becomes ingrained not only in the lives of consumers, but in the belly of corporations, we will need to be vigilant. It's MD Revolution's job to ensure that an individual's health data is protected, even from the people who are paying for it. It's our job, as digital citizens, to ensure that we monitor how corporations use our health data.

Knocking down the walls

The digital health revolution is a boon for consumers, ordinary people like myself who have limited medical knowledge. I've learned a tremendous amount about my own body by using tools like Fitbit, MyFitnessPal, and 23andMe. But it's not just consumers who benefit from these technologies. Doctors are also learning a lot from digital health.

Dr. Damani is a highly qualified cardiologist, yet he told me that he's learned more from digital health in the past year than in his entire career to date! Dr. Damani listed his impressive qualifications: "I've got a doctorate in pharmacy. I've got a doctorate in medicine. I'm board certified in internal medicine and cardiology. I've got a masters in clinical investigation. I've published over 40 papers ..." He paused dramatically. "But I'll tell you, in the last year I've learned more about how to be healthy than I've done in the previous seventeen years. And it's because I learned to measure things." As an example he cited what he's learned about how carbohydrates affect the body, by discovering more about basic nutrition and testing that knowledge with a combination of tools like MyFitnessPal, DigiFit, and Fitbit. One of his learnings: "If you want to have a high-carb meal, do it right after an interval workout, because your body's more likely to utilize it."

Dr. Damani believes that the medical fraternity is prone to over-complicating healthcare and ignoring the basic things.

How carbohydrates impact a human body is a straightforward and fundamental piece of knowledge about nutrition, yet most doctors either don't explain it to their patients or, worse, don't even know it. "There's so much that's so simple, yet we make it so complicated. Doctors sometimes aren't even equipped with that information. It's simple nutrition, but the nutritionists who are giving information are working in a silo. Just like the Fitbit is in a silo."

That word "silo", which means to operate in isolation from others, sums up much that is wrong with the healthcare system. It originated from an ancient Greek word, *siros*, which—amusingly, given how high in carbohydrates this would be—means "corn pit." One of the current definitions of silo in the *Oxford English Dictionary* is "a pit or other airtight structure in which green crops are compressed and stored as silage."

The word silo is also commonly used in the IT world, where it means a computer system, database, or even a team of people that operates in isolation from others. In the Internet landscape, silo has become synonymous with the term "walled garden," which describes an online service that allows only limited access to its information outside the official website. Facebook is a prime example. In short, both the healthcare and technology worlds are overpopulated with silos and walled gardens.

So Dr. Damani is spot-on that silos and walled gardens are preventing a lot of progress, both in digital health and the wider healthcare system. Things are slowly changing though. MD Revolution is doing its bit, chipping away at the divides. For example, MD Revolution can access much of Fitbit's data—although not all of it—but enough of Fitbit's data that it can mix it in with data from other digital health companies (23andMe, MyFitnessPal, and the like) and, crucially, its own clinical patient data.

It's only by knocking down the walled gardens and bursting open the silos that we will get a full picture of our own health. There's still a long way to go. Currently most of us don't even have access to the Electronic Medical Records housed at our family doctor's office. But MD Revolution has knocked down some of the digital health walls already. Its early users are able to mix and match, measure and monitor, their own health data.

It may be early days yet, but MD Revolution is a pointer to the future of healthcare.

EPILOGUE

The sun was on its way down as I made my way up Grant Avenue, in San Francisco's Chinatown, on a Friday afternoon in January 2013. I was on the lookout for a large "Yummy Bites" sign. This, I'd been told, was where a startup incubator called Rock Health was based. It was a strange place to locate a technology company, I mused, as I trudged up the steep street. I was used to visiting startups in downtown Palo Alto and in trendy districts of San Francisco like SoMa. I hadn't expected to find the hottest company in health technology in the middle of Chinatown.

Perhaps this sense of dislocation was preventing me from spotting the sign. I walked past it several times, as if the barrage of red and yellow colors in Chinatown had blinded me to what turned out to be a large yellow sign, jutting out into the street. I looked up to see the words "Yummy Bites" in red, Photoshopped onto a generic picture of fried rolls and noodles. It took me another 30 seconds to spot a green arrow protruding from the sign, pointing at the door. "ROCK," stated the arrow. I walked up to the door, still unconvinced that this was where the future of healthcare was being developed. The main storefront of Yummy Bites, to the left of the door, was boarded over (it had seemingly gone out of business) and the smaller window to the right was covered with blank white paper, on which had been scrawled Chinese graffiti. Below that, at foot level, was a bright yellow sign with red lettering. The words were familiar enough in that area: "Wholesale & Retail / 14k Gold / Pearl & Diamond." I looked up again at the door, which listed the present occupants of the building. I saw that Rock Health's office was on the third floor, next to Tong & Fong Accountants and below a Taoist association.

Despite its incongruous location, Rock Health is where many of Silicon Valley's health-focused startups are hatched and nurtured. Thanks to a healthy mix of Sand Hill Road venture capital money and medical establishment connections, any one of these startups might grow up to be the health equivalent of Twitter. Just as Twitter changed how we communicate, a Rock Health hatchling might end up changing the way healthcare is practiced. After all, as we've explored in this book, the medical world is being revolutionized by technology. Who knows where the next big healthcare disruptor will emerge from?

When I stepped out of the old and tiny Yummy Bites elevator onto the third floor, I saw an office space much like any other growing Silicon Valley startup: open plan, dotted with Apple computers, young and hip people milling around. It was 4:30 pm on a Friday afternoon, so I half expected the office to be emptying out for the weekend. But it was still humming with activity. A woman in her mid-twenties with long dark brown hair had noticed my entrance and waved from the other side of the office. This was Halle Tecco, the co-founder and CEO of Rock Health, and she came over to greet me. She was dressed athletically in a lemon-colored fleece sweatshirt and black stretch pants. I also noticed her long fingernails, painted navy blue. There was something of the US college sorority girl about her, with her tanned beauty and the rising inflection in her voice at the end of each sentence. But I soon discovered that despite her youth and relaxed appearance, she is one of the savviest business brains in health technology.

Over green tea in a Rock Health meeting room, Halle told me about her impressive background. She was an early starter in the world of entrepreneurship, having founded a non-profit organization in 2006 called Yoga Bear. The playful name belied a serious mission, to promote yoga to cancer patients and survivors. From the start, community was a keyword for Yoga Bear. "It's the community yoga brings," Tecco told the *Los Angeles Times* in April 2009. "The principles are all about healing and finding inner happiness, and it's a really healthy environment to be in." Tecco went on to do an MBA at Harvard Business School, starting in 2009. "I went to business school to try and figure out how I could combine my interests in healthcare and technology," she told me.

Tecco's studies culminated in a three-month internship in the summer of 2010 at the biggest technology company around: Apple. She worked in the App Store team, where her job was to review new health and medical apps for the iPhone and iPad. However, she was disappointed to find that the quality of health apps for iOS was far below that of other types of apps. At the Apple campus in Cupertino, Tecco sat next to a woman who worked with gaming developers. "She had some really awesome entrepreneurs in and out of her office all day," Tecco said. "They were building these really cool next-generation tools. But for me, in the healthcare segment, I couldn't even get some of them to upload proper images for the buttons!"

Mobile apps were all the rage in 2010, with both iPhones and Android phones selling like hot cakes. In addition, the iPad had just launched in April 2010 and there was a flurry of activity from developers over the latest magical Apple device. Yet there seemed to be very few mobile health apps worth using. MyFitnessPal, which launched its iPhone app in December 2009, was one of the rare health apps of that era to show promise. But it was an outlier. "It was sad," reflected Tecco, "because healthcare is really important. It touches all of us, but it's in a crisis. And I thought, why aren't good entrepreneurs—talented product people—working in the space?" She determined to do something about it.

Tecco started batting ideas around with a fellow MBA student at Harvard, medical student Nate Gross. "We were trying to explore why healthcare was so closed to outsiders," Tecco explained. "We learned a couple of things. One is that there are a lot of perceived barriers to healthcare, from the regulatory environment to HIPAA compliance to long sales cycles at hospitals." Those barriers made it less appealing to entrepreneurs than other industries with comparatively few barriers, like the gaming industry. "But also," continued

Tecco, "there's just, like, this old guard in healthcare. It's an industry that is set on hierarchies and degrees and resumes. It's completely the opposite of technology, which is a meritocracy." In technology, it's OK to fail—as long as you try something new. The problem was, said Tecco with a sigh, "by nature, you can't fail in healthcare." In order to try to bridge the innovation gap, Tecco and Gross decided that a startup incubator was the way to go. Both had extensive contacts and experience in the medical world, so they would be able to assist and guide new entrepreneurs to enter the healthcare industry.

Rock Health was founded as soon as Tecco's time at Apple was up, in August 2010. After a short gestation, it launched to the world in March 2011 at South by Southwest, the popular tech conference in Austin, Texas. Tecco had managed to gather an impressive list of venture capitalists behind Rock Health to provide the financing, including early Facebook investor Accel Partners. Just as important were the links to the healthcare industry, including a partnership with a leading US hospital, the Mayo Clinic.

Omada Health

Omada Health was a member of Rock Health's first class in 2011. Founded by a trio of well-educated young men, the startup set its sights on what it termed "preventable chronic disease," things like type 2 diabetes, heart disease, and stroke. According to founding CEO Sean Duffy, Omada Health was conceived while he and co-founder Adrian James were working at design consultancy IDEO. The pair had been charged with finding digital solutions to disease prevention. Just as Martin Blinder, the founder of health dashboard TicTrac (profiled in Chapter Eight) had done, Sean Duffy and Adrian James soon left their consultant jobs to spin off one of their ideas as a startup. They were joined by a third co-founder, Andrew DiMichele. Rock Health had just launched, so the trio applied for and were accepted into the first class. By the end of 2012, Omada Health had launched to the public.

In a sense, Omada Health is an amalgam of all of the themes I've written about in this book. It's trying to help its users make lifestyle changes in order to improve their health. To do this it not only provides self-tracking tools, but also emphasizes social support by putting users into small groups based on BMI (Body Mass Index), age, and location. Finally, Omada Health provides a "Health Coach" to guide the participants, similar to what MD Revolution (the subject of the previous chapter) does.

Omada Health is focusing on type 2 diabetes first, citing statistical evidence that "prediabetes currently affects 79 million people in the US and over 1 billion worldwide." Its debut service is called "Prevent" and is a sixteen-week online program that primarily helps people at risk of type 2 diabetes to lose weight. At $120 per month, the program is not cheap. But that price includes a WiFi scale and pedometer. The program starts with changing your food habits, with the help of self-tracking tools to monitor your food intake and weight. The next step is to increase your activity level, using the "Prevent pedometer" to track this. You're also given a weekly activity goal, which you're encouraged to meet "with the support and effort of your Prevent group members." The last phase is about sustaining these lifestyle changes, through continued social support and setting ongoing goals.

Like MD Revolution, Omada Health is at its heart a support system for using self-tracking tools and techniques. It's less clinically focused than MD Revolution and more akin to a Weight Watchers program. Indeed, a key similarity to Weight Watchers is that Omada's "Health Coaches" often come from the ranks of its former participants. The coaches are paid based on performance, so there is a possible financial as well as health incentive to do the program.

Also like Weight Watchers, Omada Health cites clinical research to back up its methods. The Prevent program is based on the results of the Diabetes Prevention Program (DPP) clinical trial, an initiative of the National Institutes of Health (NIH). The trial found that "participants who lost a modest amount of weight through dietary changes and increased physical activity sharply reduced their chances of developing diabetes." Significantly, this was compared to the traditional method of taking drugs to ward off disease: "DPP participants who took the oral diabetes medication metformin also reduced their risk of developing diabetes, but not as much as those in the lifestyle intervention group." These findings were published in February 2002 in the *New England Journal of Medicine*.

Of course, as we've discovered in this book, the alternative to paying Omada Health $120 per month is to do it all yourself—for free. You can track your food, activity, weight, and other measures using tools like MyFitnessPal. However, as we've also learned, lifestyle change is hard. Just ask Buster Benson, the ultimate self-tracker (profiled in Chapter One). Having a support system is vital to the success of self-tracking and that's what Omada Health (and MD Revolution) bring to the table.

Halle Tecco is justifiably proud of the success of her Rock Health graduates, such as Omada Health. But does she self-track herself, I asked? She pointed to a bracelet on her wrist, which turned out to be a Jawbone UP. Similar to a Fitbit, the UP tracks how many steps you take in a day. However, I sensed that Tecco was kind of blasé about the device. "It's fine, but ..." she paused to find the right words, in order to break it to me gently. "Tracking isn't what gets me really excited about healthcare. Changing behavior does."

Tecco doesn't just mean people changing their lifestyles. She wants the healthcare system to change *its* behavior too. "It's really important that we all have transparency to healthcare cost," she explained. "That we know, before going to the hospital, how much it's going to cost. Or if it's cheaper down the road." Halle Tecco paused and turned her attention back to the UP bracelet on her wrist. She lifted her arm and gave the bracelet a bit of a jangle. "But I think that this is a really great gateway drug," she laughed, "to get people excited about healthcare."

> "It's really important that we all have transparency to healthcare cost."

Who will pay for it?

Throughout this book I've emphasized that creating a better healthcare system will need both the medical establishment to change its old ways, and individuals to take more responsibility for their own health. But there is an elephant in the room, and Halle Tecco pointed it out. "I think our biggest challenge is reimbursement or payment for direct-to-consumer products," she said. In other words, although people can easily track their own health nowadays, there is a cost to it.

A Fitbit will help you be more active, and results in improved health. But the device costs around $100. For many people, that's too expensive. Even free apps, such as MyFitnessPal, require a smartphone to run on—and while those are getting cheaper, there will always be a telecommunications company to pay each month.

Tecco believes it comes down to the insurance companies. If they would pay a relatively small amount for a device or app that helps you avoid getting type 2 diabetes, in the long run that's a lot cheaper than paying for your doctor and specialist visits. "The insurer has incentives to want this because this is cheaper and just as effective," Tecco explained. "The insurance companies need to become more active in recognizing when they should reimburse for things." However, Tecco acknowledges this is a tough sell to insurance companies. "Even if they could save money, even if you eat healthy and work out every day, which saves your insurance company lots of money down the road, they're not going to pay for it now," she said, shaking her head dolefully. What she means is that insurance companies are already paying for doctors to treat you, so paying for self-tracking devices on top of that cuts into their short-term bottom line.

There is a stalemate situation among the three players: the medical establishment, health insurance companies, and consumers. Nobody wants to lose money or pay it out. But prominent health technology investor Esther Dyson thinks she has a solution. She has set up a community initiative called HICCup, the Health Intervention Coordinating Council. It will help communities adopt healthier lifestyles without having to deal with insurance companies or even the medical establishment. In a manifesto published in May 2013, Dyson wrote:

> *It is hard to find anyone in healthcare who does not believe that spending $100 now on healthy behavior— exercise and proper nutrition, counseling for pre-diabetics, risk monitoring, and so on—could yield more than $200 in reduced costs and improved outcomes later … And yet neither individuals nor communities seem to act on the basis of this knowledge.*

Dyson set up HICCup to tackle this problem. She describes it as "a self-appointed counseling service aimed at persuading local institutions to embrace a long-term perspective and launch a full-scale intervention in their communities." The organization is initially focusing on several communities of 100,000 people or fewer. Dyson is aiming for small changes in everyday health in these communities, such as implementing healthier school lunch options or encouraging people to walk more. HICCup's self-described "counselors" will work with community leaders and advocates to bring about these changes.

Dyson's project is all about making incremental improvements to health and preventing disease. She admits though that even this comes down to cost. In the manifesto, Dyson appealed for "a benevolent but ultimately profit-driven billionaire or hedge fund" to bankroll the initiative. Regardless of whether she finds her Bill Gates or Warren Buffett, Dyson acknowledges that technology has at least paved the way. "A lot of this requires very little exotic technology," she told MIT's *Technology Review* magazine in September 2013. "What it requires is social buy-in and changes in diet. But technology can help because it's a reminder, it's personal, and it's cheap."

This isn't all about doing good in the world for Dyson. She has a good deal of skin in the game too. Her day job is angel investor, with a particular focus on health technology startups. She was a first-round investor in Omada Health, the Rock Health-incubated startup I discussed earlier. She was also one of the first investors in 23andMe and is on its board of directors. Dyson is very open about having profit motives as well as wanting to help communities. The HICCup website notes that its two biggest challenges are "to help people (stay) healthy, and to change the system so that at least some of the cost savings of a healthier population can be captured by investors who fund the changes upfront. (Otherwise, why would they invest?)"

Ultimately, Dyson wants to "let communities choose which technologies and interventions they want to use." Of course, she wouldn't mind if they chose the startups she invested in. But her investment philosophy is to put money into the type of health startup that will make a difference in the community. "There are devices to tell you how many steps you took, the composition of the blood, and sleep patterns," she told *Technology Review*. "Those are more personal, they are more self-involving if they are well designed, [and] they can be gamified so that you just want those extra points, and you'll take another walk around the block in order to get them."

It's too early to say whether Esther Dyson's HICCup initiative will even get off the ground, let alone create healthier communities. There are as yet no details about which communities she is targeting, or what specific projects will be undertaken. But there is something refreshing about her approach: that communities can drive this change and we don't necessarily need the medical establishment or insurance companies on board.

Although a big theme of this book is self-reliance and taking responsibility for your own health, it's going to take more than that to improve health at a population level. As the HICCup website proclaims: "We believe that you can't really induce or preserve health one person at a time; there needs to be environmental change. Just as our surroundings make us sick, so can they keep us healthy."

Buster Benson's resolution

I began this book by profiling Buster Benson, a former Seattle resident in his mid-thirties who now works for Twitter in San

Francisco. There are few people in the world today who are more dedicated to self-tracking than Benson. He not only self-tracks to improve his health—the main focus of this book—but also to create better daily habits, to search for meaning in his life, and to find happiness. "Dedicated" is the kindest way to describe him. Some would call him obsessed. That said, let's check in on Buster Benson and see how he's getting on with his 2013 tracking goals.

Benson's primary goal at the beginning of 2013 was to become more proactive first thing in the morning, which he thought might improve his morning habits and ultimately make him happier. He wrote it down as a New Year's resolution on January 1: "At least 5 days a week, start my day proactively by doing at least one of these 6 things before looking at my phone: drink a glass of water, stretch, do pushups, do lunges, do plank, review my haiku deck." He recorded this resolution in a Google Groups forum he set up, playfully entitled "Rabbit Rabbit Resolution Accountability Squad," inviting his friends and Twitter acquaintances to do the same.

The idea with the forum was that everyone would do a public "check-in" on the first day of every month to update fellow participants on their progress. As the name of the group suggested, this brought a certain accountability to the self-tracking that each person would do.

At the time I interviewed Benson for this book, toward the end of January 2013, he was struggling with the resolution. He'd recently moved his young family down to San Francisco and, he told me, there were too many real-world distractions for him to focus on being proactive early in the mornings. Sure enough, in his February 1 check-in he graded himself badly for January. "According to my Lift app," he wrote (referring to a journaling iPhone app popular in Silicon Valley at the time), "I only did this 12 out of the 31 days in January. I continue to learn how much I am not a morning person." However, now that he and his family were settled in San Francisco, he determined to keep going with the resolution. He wrote: "We're now in San Francisco, have a new place, and our lives are much more predictable. I think it's a perfect time to renew my resolution."

He made a few modifications though, removing lunges and plank from the six options of things to do before looking at his phone in the morning. In its place was a new option: "Hold my breath and meditate as long as I can."

Come March 1 and Benson had finally settled into the early morning resolution. He commented that "the most rewarding part of this routine is the drinking of water, remembering my 'memento mori' list [his haiku deck], and stretching." For the coming month, he resolved to "be more specific about the morning routine and try to stick to it for the full month."

The April 1 check-in was even more positive: "This is the first month that I felt like I found my stride. I only missed two days. And also, found that the morning routine was a part of the day that I looked forward to." He renewed the same resolution for the coming month, noting that "I don't think I've ever had a resolution that I still actively thought about in April."

However, by May 1 there were signs that Benson's New Year's resolution was no longer satisfying for him. He changed it from an early morning routine to a more general daily resolve to "meditate for at least five minutes a day, at least six days a week." No more "6 options" before breakfast; now it was just about meditating for five short minutes a day.

Jumping ahead a couple of months to July 1, by this point Benson had clearly tired of the resolution. He admitted that he'd become obsessed with "streaks"—doing a certain thing every day until the continuity was broken due to travel or another factor that disrupted his routine. He resolved to scale back his self-tracking for the coming month: "No more going for streaks in Lift or Equanimity [a meditation timer and tracker app]. The overhead is just too much for me and is a bit too stressful."

By August 1, Buster had decided to change tack and focus on something completely different. He resolved to "to track at least 5 'quality times' a week." By quality time, he meant time spent with his wife Kellianne, son Niko, himself, and his work.

Tellingly, he added at the end of his August 1 update: "Also, I've been sick for 2 weeks and just need to get better."

On September 1 Benson checked in again. But unfortunately, he hadn't succeeded in the new resolution either. This time he blamed travel and the nebulousness of what "quality time" meant. Somewhat mournfully, he declared that "I'm on a miss streak." The past few months had all been marked as a "MISS" in terms of the goals he'd set himself.

So in the space of seven months, Buster Benson's New Year's resolution had fizzled out—like so many resolutions that people make on January 1.

What went wrong with Buster's self-tracking resolutions throughout 2013? He had begun with a noble resolution to be more proactive first thing in the morning. When I interviewed Buster at the end of January, I'd seen signs that his resolution might be tough going. But it got better in February and then again in March and April. However, after that it seems like he quickly tired of the daily grind of meeting his resolution. Reflecting on this, Buster wrote at the end of August: "Goals, habits, and resolutions are often crafted with ambitious expectations that are then susceptible to the first rainy day, sick day, vacation day, holiday, grumpy day, low-energy day, or otherwise non-standard day." What happened to his resolution, he concluded, was what he ruefully termed "Life's Chaos Monkey." He meant that the unpredictable nature of our daily life often derails our attempts at behavior change.

Despite the setbacks, Buster continues to tinker and experiment with his self-tracking methods—just as he always will. As I write this, his latest theory is to track his "modes" of living. I won't describe what that is here, because I'm willing to bet he will have moved onto yet another new theory in a few months. Yet I don't consider Buster Benson fickle or changeable when it comes to his self-tracking. In fact, I admire him for trying new things and constantly looking for ways to improve himself. That's ultimately what being a self-tracker is all about: experimenting with new ways of living, and seeing whether they work.

My self-tracking year

As I look back on my own experience of self-tracking this year, I realize that it's not too dissimilar to Buster's experience. That is, things changed. Life happened and I adjusted what I tracked accordingly.

I used Fitbit for several months earlier this year, dutifully attaching the device to my belt every day and tracking my daily steps. A couple of times I thought I'd lost the little device, once when I was down in Wanaka, a beautiful area of the South Island of New Zealand, for a conference. I'd gone for a trek up a scenic hill with fellow conference attendees, only to discover to my dismay at the top of the hill that my Fitbit had disappeared. Funnily enough, my first thought was *not* that I'd just lost a device that cost $100—but that I wouldn't get the credit for all those steps I'd just climbed! Happily, I recovered the device on the trip back to the conference venue. One of my fellow trekkers had picked it up on the way down the hill. I was still cross that I'd missed logging those hard-earned steps though.

Soon after I got back home, I stopped using Fitbit, not because I wasn't happy with the product, but because I'd found out what I needed to know. It had served its purpose at that time in my life. It had made me more aware of how little activity I do in a day if I don't go out for a walk, even if only to the café. On a good day I averaged around 8,000 steps, a bit below the 10,000 steps per day mark that has become the de facto definition of "active." But for me, 8,000 steps was active enough.

I also stopped using Fitbit because I discovered that the foods I consumed were a more important marker for health. So I switched my focus to tracking my food, using the MyFitnessPal iPhone app. Because I'm a type 1 diabetic, my main daily health concern is controlling my blood sugar levels. I'd found out that although my daily activity was important for my sense of wellbeing, it didn't really have much impact on my blood sugar levels. What did was a big change in March of 2013, when I started on a low-carbohydrate diet. During this period I closely monitored my daily food intake on MyFitnessPal, paying particular attention to the amount of carbohydrates I consumed. For a while I cross-checked this with my Fitbit activity data, often using the TicTrac dashboard to compare the two sets of data.

I stopped using MyFitnessPal too, after a few months. By that time I'd settled into a fairly regular eating routine, so I didn't feel like I needed to continue tracking it. More important, through using MyFitnessPal for a few months and closely monitoring my data, I had learned to accurately estimate my daily carbohydrate intake so that I didn't need to input everything. I'm pretty sure I'll go back and use Fitbit and MyFitnessPal again, for further two- or three-month stints. Self-tracking, when it comes down to it, is all about understanding what's happening in your body and mind at a certain period of time. And life constantly changes. Your circumstances shift from time to time and the "chaos monkey" (to use Buster Benson's term) meddles in your life every now and then. So when those changes happen, I may want to measure and monitor how it impacts on my health. I may also want to see how different seasons affect me, for example by tracking my Fitbit data over a summer and winter and comparing my activity levels.

There are many different reasons to track various aspects of your life— your activity, food intake, weight, daily mood, blood sugar levels, heart rate … the list goes on. But I learned that you don't need to be obsessive about it. Track when you want to know something about your body or mind. Then don't track it. You can always come back to it again later.

Self-tracking is all about understanding what's happening in your body and mind at a certain period of time.

It's also worth noting that as new technology comes onto the market, self-tracking will become more seamless. Apple is betting on people wearing its Apple Watch all day and every day. In this scenario, health data is collected routinely by the watch and without you necessarily noticing. The benefit of this is that tracking happens in the background and you'll only check it when you need to.

The most troublesome aspect of this book was the subject that has had the most media attention, by far, of all the topics I've covered: personal genomics. I did a 23andMe test in 2012 and I was happy with the things I learned, such as my increased genetic risk of getting type 1 diabetes. But I struggled to find any practical use for my DNA data. Even if I'd found out about my increased risk before I was diagnosed with type 1 in November 2007, there was nothing I could have done to prevent it. That's the key issue that 23andMe and the entire genetics industry is grappling with currently: how to make use of this data. In terms of self-tracking, your DNA will always stay the same so you only need to "track" it once. However, your microbiome—the creatures that your body plays host to—will change over time. So doing a regular test with a company like uBiome may become a factor in self-tracking in the future.

However self-tracking pans out, I'm certain that it will produce data that is of interest to, and is used by, your doctor and the medical establishment as a whole. You have the ability to manage your health and prevent certain diseases (like type 2 diabetes) more easily now by using tracking tools. I must stress that it will never replace the experts—your doctor and medical professionals. Their role in your health, however, will change. It will shift from a focus on treating you when you're sick to helping you prevent sickness in the first place. As Dr. Robin Berzin, the New York City doctor I profiled in Chapter Nine, put it:

> The notion of what it means to be healthy is changing
> for most of us. It's no longer just about not being sick, or
> not having a disease with a name, like cancer or diabetes
> or high blood pressure. Today, health is more than that.
> Health is vitality, energy, a sense of calm, and a body that
> doesn't hold you back. A body that is your vehicle in life,
> firing on all cylinders and ready to take you where you
> want to go. It's not about looking perfect. It's about feeling
> supple, strong, and light on your feet, whatever your
> weight happens to be.

Whether you track your daily vitality on your own (whenever you need to), or whether you enlist the help of your doctor or new types of healthcare services like MD Revolution and Omada Health, it all comes back to your personal wellbeing. The difference is that now you don't need a doctor to tell you what to do. By becoming a tracker, you can manage much of your daily healthcare by yourself.

THE AUTHOR

Richard MacManus is the founder of technology blog ReadWrite. com. Widely read globally, it focused on the US market and was syndicated by *The New York Times* from 2008 to 2011. In 2011, Richard sold ReadWrite to San Francisco-based SAY Media and in 2012 left his job there as Editor-in-Chief to write this, his first book. As ReadWrite's founder, he is widely recognized as a leader in articulating what's next in technology and what it means for society at large. He became interested in health technology when diagnosed with type 1 diabetes and he has written many articles about consumer health products and trends.

Richard's homepage is http://ricm.ac. He is active on social media and you can follow his ongoing thoughts about self-tracking on Facebook and Twitter, under the handle @ricmac. Richard lives in Wellington, New Zealand.

FURTHER READING
& REFERENCES

Aljasir B, Bryson M & Al-shehri B. "Yoga Practice for the Management of Type II Diabetes Mellitus in Adults: A systematic Review" in *Evidence-Based Complementary and Alternative Medicine*, vol. 7, (4)399–408, 2010

Atkins, Robert C. *Dr. Atkins' Diet Revolution: The High Calorie Way to Stay Thin Forever*, D. McKay Co, New York, 1972

Bassett Jr, David R & Strath, Scott J. "Use of pedometers to assess physical activity" in *Physical Activity Assessments for Health-Related Research*, Human Kinetics, Champaign, Illinois, 2002

Bernstein, Richard K. *Dr. Bernstein's Diabetes Solution: The Complete Guide to Achieving Normal Blood Sugars*, Little, Brown and Company, New York, 2007

Carey, Nessa. *The Epigenetics Revolution: How Modern Biology Is Rewriting Our Understanding of Genetics, Disease, and Inheritance*, Columbia University Press, New York, 2012

da Vinci, Leonardo (trans. Richter, Jean Paul). *The Notebooks of Leonardo Da Vinci*, http://en.wikisource.org/wiki/The_Notebooks_of_Leonardo_Da_Vinci

Gibbs-Smith, Charles H & Rees, Gareth. *The Inventions of Leonardo Da Vinci*, Peerage/ Scribner Book Company, New York, 1978

Gladwell, Malcolm. *Outliers: The Story of Success*, Little, Brown and Company, New York, 2007

Heshka S, Anderson JW, Atkinson RL, Greenway FL, Hill JO, Phinney SD, Kolotkin RL, Miller-Kovach K & Pi-Sunyer FX. "Weight loss with self-help compared with a structured commercial program: a randomized trial" in *JAMA. Journal of the American Medical Association*, 289(14):1792–8, April 9, 2003

Hölzel BK, Carmody J, Vangel M, Congleton C, Yerramsetti SM, Gard T, Lazar SW. "Mindfulness practice leads to increases in regional brain gray matter density" in *Psychiatry Research: Neuroimaging* 191, Elsevier, 2011

Hsiao, Chun-Ju & Hing, Esther. "Use and Characteristics of Electronic Health Record Systems Among Office-based Physician Practices: United States, 2001–2012" in *NCHS Data Brief*, National Center for Health Statistics, Number 111, December 2012

Jefferson, Thomas (ed. Peterson, Merrill D). *Thomas Jefferson: Writings : Autobiography / Notes on the State of Virginia / Public and Private Papers / Addresses / Letters (Library of America)*, Library of America, New York, 1984

Jobson, Ross W. & Antell, Peter M. *President's Council on Fitness, Sports & Nutrition: The First 50 Years: 1956–2006*, Tampa, Florida, 2006

Knowler WC, Barrett-Connor E, Fowler SE, Hamman RF, Lachin JM, Walker EA, & Nathan DM; Diabetes Prevention Program Research Group. "Reduction in the Incidence of Type 2 Diabetes with Lifestyle Intervention or Metformin" in the *New England Journal of Medicine* 346:393–403, February 7, 2002

Mukherjee, Siddhartha. *The Emperor of All Maladies: A Biography of Cancer*, Scribner, New York, 2010

Nidetch, Jean. *The Story of Weight Watchers*, Signet, New York, 1979

Ohta, Dr. T. "Shadow of Buddhism and Shintoism in neurosurgical practice in Japan" in *Medical Technologies in Neurosurgery*, (eds. Nimsky, Christopher & Fahlbusch, Rudolf), SpringerWien, New York, 2006

Pritikin, Nathan. *Pritikin Program for Diet and Exercise*, Putnam Pub Group, New York, 1982

"Probiotics Market by Products (Functional Foods, Dietary Supplements, Specialty Nutrients, Animal Feed), Applications (Regular, Therapeutic, Preventive Health Care) & Ingredients (Lactobacilli, Bifidobacteria, Yeast)—Global Trends & Forecasts to 2019" report March 2014, http://Marketsandmarkets.com

Relman, David A. "Microbiology: Learning about who we are" in *Nature* 486, 194–195, June 14, 2012

Ruhl, Jenny. *Diet 101: The Truth About Low Carb Diets*, Technion Books, Turners Falls, Massachusetts, 2012

Stone, Judy. "uBiome: Ethical Lapse or Not?" in Scientific American Blog Network, July 25, 2013, http://blogs.scientificamerican.com/molecules-to-medicine/2013/07/25/ubiome-ethical-lapse-or-not/

Taubes, Gary. 'What if It's All Been a Big Fat Lie?' *New York Times*, July 7, 2002

Taubes, Gary. *Good Calories, Bad Calories: Challenging the Conventional Wisdom on Diet, Weight Control, and Disease*, Knopf, New York, 2007

The Wellcome Trust Case Control Consortium. "Genome-wide association study of 14,000 cases of seven common diseases and 3,000 shared controls" in *Nature*, 447(7145): 661–6787, June 2007

Topol, Eric. *The Creative Destruction of Medicine: How the Digital Revolution Will Create Better Health Care*, Basic Books, New York, 2012

Tudor-Locke C, Hatano Y, Pangrazi RP & Kang M. "Revisiting 'how many steps are enough?'" in *Medicine and Science in Sports and Exercise*, vol. 40, issue 7, July 2008

Tudor-Locke, Catrine & Bassett Jr, David R. "How Many Steps/Day Are Enough?: Preliminary Pedometer Indices for Public Health" in *Sports Medicine*, vol. 34, issue 1, 2004

Williams, Ulric. *Hints on Healthy Living*, South's Book Depot, Wellington, 1935

INDEX

10,000 steps (a day) 50–54, 55, 123, 188, 191, 214
23andMe 14, 18, 19, 22, 38, 96, 97–114, 129, 131, 132, 133, 137, 138–140, 143, 144, 146, 173, 185, 189, 192, 193, 199, 200, 210, 216

Alzheimer's disease 102, 103, 109, 113, 123
American Diabetes Association (ADA) 69, 91
American Heart Association (AHA) 69
Android/s 15, 16, 65, 66, 159, 204
Apple Watch 16, 24, 58, 215
Application Programing Interface (APIs) 159–162
Apte, Dr. Zachary 131
Atkins diet, the, *see* Atkins, Dr. Robert
Atkins, Dr. Robert 62, 63, 64, 65, 69, 70, 71, 72, 75, 89
autoimmune diseases 20, 170, 178
Avey, Linda 96, 102, 103
Ayurveda 169–170

Bates, Dr. Melissa 136, 137
Beacon 158, 159, 161
behavior change 21, 32, 33, 93, 171, 194, 196, 197, 213
Benson, Buster 21, 23–40, 189, 196, 207, 210, 215
Berzin, Dr. Robin 19, 22, 154, 166–183, 189, 216
Blinder, Martin 147, 148–150, 151, 152, 153, 154, 155, 156, 157, 162, 165, 205
blood pressure 13, 57, 71, 147,

148, 152, 153, 154, 162, 175, 176, 185, 191, 216
body fat percentage 82
body mass index (BMI) 75, 81, 83, 84, 198, 206
brain docks 121–123
brain imaging 117
brain scans 14, 21, 120, 123, 124, 126, 127
Brainstorm Research Foundation 102

calorie counting 60, 61, 64, 65, 66, 69, 70, 74, 75, 91, 93
cancer 20, 81, 108, 170, 178, 203, 216
citizen science 135, 143
complementary medicine 168
crowdfunding 129, 131, 132, 135
crowdsourcing 68, 138–142
Curious 101, 102, 103, 104, 193

Damani, Dr. Samir 22, 184, 185, 186, 187, 188, 189, 190, 191, 192, 193, 194, 195, 197, 198, 199, 200
dashboard/s 93, 138, 142, 147–165, 184, 186, 188, 190, 191, 193, 195, 198, 205, 215. *See also* RevUp, TicTrac
da Vinci, Leonardo 54, 55
deCODE genetics 96, 98
diabetes 9, 10, 11, 12, 13, 14, 18, 20, 21, 50, 75, 76, 81, 96, 97, 99, 100, 101, 105, 107, 108, 109, 110, 111, 112, 113, 168, 169, 174, 179, 180, 181, 192, 205, 206, 207, 208, 216. *See also* diabetic/s
diabetic/s 13, 72, 75, 91, 96, 110, 133, 173, 174, 179, 180, 181, 182,

209, 214. *See also* diabetes

diet/s/dieting 12, 13, 51, 53, 60, 61–65, 69–73, 74, 75, 76, 78, 79, 84, 88, 89, 90, 94, 133, 143, 145, 168, 179, 180, 181, 186, 188, 209, 214. *See also* Atkins, Dr. Robert; Pritikin, Dr. Nathan; Paleo diet

DNA 18, 19, 20, 22, 38, 96, 97, 98, 100, 101, 105, 107, 108, 110, 129, 131, 132, 146, 186, 188, 192, 194, 216

Dyson, Esther 208, 209, 210

electroconvulsive therapy (ECT) 121

Electronic Health/Medical Record (EHR/EMR) 162, 163, 164, 165, 172, 173, 194, 195

enterotypes 133

epigenetics 108–111, 112. *See also* genetics; personal genomics

Facebook 30, 68, 85, 102, 143, 151, 155, 156, 157, 158, 160, 161, 171, 191, 200, 205

FDA (US Food & Drug Administration) 67, 101, 137, 162

Fitbit 14, 17, 19, 20, 21, 24, 41–58, 65, 66, 73, 78, 82, 89, 117, 123, 125, 130, 138, 143, 144, 145, 146, 149, 152, 153, 159, 160, 173, 175, 177, 179, 182, 184, 185, 188, 189, 190, 191, 193, 195, 196, 197, 199, 200, 207, 208, 214, 215

food intake 66, 70, 72, 73, 75, 91, 93, 146, 169, 206, 214, 215

food tracking 51, 61, 65, 67, 73, 74, 91, 186

Friedlander, Robin *see* Berzin, Dr. Robin

Friedman, Eric 41, 42, 43, 44, 45, 46, 47, 48, 49, 50, 53, 54, 56, 58

gamification 30, 189

genetics 38, 96–114, 138, 139, 142, 187, 188, 191, 216

genome/s 38, 96, 97, 98, 100, 102, 104, 108, 129, 130, 133, 134, 140, 141. *See also* genetics; personal genomics

genotype/s 100, 102, 103, 107, 109, 193

Glycemic Index (GI) 69, 70, 132

Goh, Crystal 115, 116, 117, 118, 119, 120, 121, 123, 124, 125, 126, 127

Google 16, 32, 87, 96, 97, 100, 131, 139, 144, 150, 151, 155, 156, 161, 184, 211

Greenhall, Amelia 15, 21, 78, 79, 80, 81, 86, 87, 88, 89, 93, 94, 95, 152

Health Month 29, 30, 32

health technology 9, 65, 123, 130, 138, 153, 182, 183, 202, 203, 208, 209

heart disease 20, 52, 62, 63, 81, 104, 105, 106, 107, 112, 168, 170, 178, 205

heart rate 14, 182, 183, 186, 188, 193, 194, 198, 215

HICCup (Health Intervention Coordinating Council) 208, 209, 210

HITECH 164, 194

human genome, *see* genome/s

Human Microbiome Project 129, 140, 141

iCalorie 16–17

iGoogle 150, 151, 153, 161
immune system 12, 110, 129
Indiegogo, *see* crowdfunding
integrative medicine 166, 167–168, 169, 173, 179, 183
iPad 13, 14, 19, 159, 163, 164, 176, 204
iPhone 11, 14, 16, 17, 37, 57, 65, 66, 73, 148, 156, 159, 175, 176, 204, 211, 214

Jawbone UP 56, 58, 207
Jefferson, Thomas 54, 55
Jobs, Steve 135, 176

Kickstarter, *see* crowdfunding

Lee, Mike 28, 59, 60, 61, 65, 66, 67, 68, 73, 74, 75, 76, 77
lifestyle 20, 21, 22, 24, 29, 33, 36, 52, 53, 56, 79, 80, 81, 87, 88, 94, 104, 109, 119, 120, 122, 123, 145, 146, 154, 165, 168, 178, 206, 207
Ludington, Dr. Will 131

MacCarthy, Oliver 150, 151, 152
macrobiotic diet 168
MD Revolution 22, 184–200, 201, 206, 207, 217
meditation 120, 124, 125, 126, 168, 169, 181, 212
microbiome 103, 128–146, 216
Microsoft 26, 43, 150, 151
Miller-Kovach, Karen 90, 91, 92, 93
Morale-O-Meter 24, 29
MRI (magnetic resonance imaging) 115, 117, 118, 123, 124, 125, 126, 127
MyFitnessPal 14, 17, 20, 22, 24, 28, 59–77, 85, 93, 138, 144, 145, 146, 173, 175, 177, 179, 184, 185, 186,

188, 189, 191, 193, 195, 196, 197, 199, 200, 204, 207, 208, 214, 215
National Institutes of Health (NIH) 129, 140, 142, 206
Navigenics 96, 98
neuroplasticity 120
Neuroprofile 115, 117–120, 121, 123, 126, 127
neuroscience 115, 117, 123, 124, 125, 126
Nidetch, Jean 84, 88, 89, 90
Nike 24, 32, 46, 56, 58, 73
ningen dock, *see* brain docks
nutrition 17, 53, 67, 68, 111, 189, 191, 193, 199, 200, 209

obese 71, 81, 82, 83, 84, 93, 180, 192. *See also* obesity
obesity 71, 82, 83, 94, 168, 169, 180, 193. *See also* obese
Omada Health 204–206, 207, 209, 217
Oz, Dr. Mehmet 166, 167, 168, 171

Paleo diet 71, 72
Park, James 41, 42, 43, 44, 45, 46, 47, 48, 49, 50, 53
Parkinson's disease 113, 139, 140
PDA 59, 60
Pebble watch 24
pedometers 14, 17, 24, 41, 42, 44, 45, 46, 50, 52, 54, 55, 56, 58, 73, 78, 123, 206
personal genomics 14, 18, 20, 21, 97, 98, 162, 192, 194, 216. *See also* genetics, genomes
phenotype/s 102, 103, 193
PointsPlus 92, 93
Pollock, James 152
preventative medicine 20, 107, 170

Pritikin diet, the, *see* Pritikin, Dr.
  Nathan
Pritikin, Dr. Nathan 63, 64, 69, 75
privacy 142, 157–159, 194, 195,
  197, 199
probiotic 134, 137

quantified self 15, 25, 36, 119, 138

RevUp 184, 186, 188, 189, 191–
  194, 195, 198
Richman, Jessica 128, 129, 130,
  131, 133, 134, 135, 136, 137, 139,
  140, 142, 143, 144, 146
Rock Health 202, 203, 205, 207, 209

self-tracking 14, 15, 16, 17, 20, 21,
  22, 23, 24, 25, 26, 27, 28, 30, 31,
  32, 33, 34, 35, 36, 37, 38, 39, 40,
  53, 57, 58, 79, 87, 93, 94, 95, 98,
  137, 142, 143, 145, 146, 152, 168,
  170, 171, 173, 175, 176, 186, 189,
  191, 196, 197, 198, 199, 206, 207,
  208, 211, 212, 213, 214, 215, 216
single nucleotide polymorphisms
  (SNPs) 98, 99, 100, 101, 105
smartphone 13, 16, 17, 18, 24, 60,
  65, 73, 76, 144, 171, 176, 184,
  186, 208
smart watch 58. *See also* Apple
  Watch, Pebble watch
SNPedia 99, 100
social support 21, 33, 81, 84, 86,
  196, 197, 206
Stone, Dr. Judy 135, 136, 137, 139,
  142
stress 10, 12, 88, 113, 125, 147,
  148, 152, 153, 154, 165, 216

Taubes, Gary 70, 71, 75
Tecco, Halle 203, 204, 205, 207, 208

TechCrunch 50 48, 56
TicTrac 142, 147–165, 184, 191,
  192, 194, 195, 205, 215
Twitter 13, 26, 27, 31, 68, 130, 143,
  149, 155, 160, 171, 203, 210

uBiome 128–146, 173, 216

vegetarian/ism 33, 64, 72, 79, 94,
  168
VO2 188

wearable devices 21, 43, 57
Wearable Internet 56
weight loss 21, 64, 71, 78, 83, 84,
  86, 93, 142
weight tracking 78–95
Weight Watchers 21, 33, 70,
  81–87, 88, 89–93, 94, 95, 196,
  197, 206
wellness 14, 48, 58, 120, 162–165,
  195, 197, 198, 199
Williams, Dr. Ulric 177, 178, 179
Withings scale 18, 24, 57, 78, 79,
  82, 89, 148, 149, 152, 160, 173,
  183, 184, 186, 189, 190, 191
Wojcicki, Anne 19, 97, 102, 138,
  139, 140
World Health Organization
  (WHO) 81, 82, 83, 84, 93

Yahoo 150, 155, 184
yoga 79, 124, 125, 168, 169, 181,
  182, 183, 203